Weight Training
for a
New Body

Over 300 Exercises to Tone, Strengthen, and Build Muscle

Mike Croskery, B.Sc. H.K., PFLC

MyoMax Performance Publications
Dunrobin, Ontario

Published by MyoMax Performance, Dunrobin, Ontario, Canada
www.myomaxfitness.com; myomax@irtech.com

Printed in Canada
First Printing March 2004
Second Printing July 2005

National Library of Canada Cataloguing in Publication

Croskery, Mike, 1972-
    Weight training for a new body : over 300 exercises to tone, strengthen and
build muscle / Mike Croskery.

Includes index.
New ed. of: The weight trainer's exercise handbook.
ISBN 0-9688365-1-8

    1. Weight training. I. Title.

GV546.C77 2004   613.7'13   C2004-901537-0

DISCLAIMER: Every attempt has been made by the author to ensure that the information in this
book is accurate. The information is intended to provide basic guidelines for weight training and
stretching exercise execution and weight training program development. Each person has
different needs, abilities, and fitness levels. Consult your physician as well as other medical and
fitness professionals before starting any exercise routine. The author does not accept any
responsibility or liability for the use or misuse of the information contained in this handbook.

Distributed by **Gordon Soules Book
Publishers Ltd.** ● 1359 Ambleside Lane,
West Vancouver, BC, Canada V7T 2Y9
● PMB 620, 1916 Pike Place #12,
Seattle, WA 98101-1097 US
E-mail: books@gordonsoules.com
Web site: http://www.gordonsoules.com
(604) 922 6588 Fax: (604) 688 5442

TABLE OF CONTENTS

TABLE OF CONTENTS

ACKNOWLEDGEMENTS

No production is a one-man show. I would like to express my appreciation and gratitude to the many people who have helped this book become what it has. From the point when I picked up my first weight to the last time I proof read this book there have been many people who have helped me along the way. When I was working on this book as a second edition to the Weight Trainer's Exercise Handbook, I listened to people who had read the book and took their advice to heart.

Without the help of my wife, Tally, there would have been no pictures and probably no second edition. Many late nights were spent taking pictures, and retaking pictures, to insure that those who chose this book as their guide would get the best visual descriptions of the exercises. Her strong support and belief in myself, and in making this book even better through countless hours of proof reading and re-editing, has helped me realize my ideas and dreams. For this and for her time, energy and sense of humour that kept me focused on this project, I extend my heartfelt thanks and am forever grateful.

My mother and editor, Lorraine Croskery, who has helped me put words together time and time again was invaluable in finalizing this book. Writing as simply and as clearly as possible is one of the most challenging factors in conveying information. Without her input this book would not be as readable as I trust it is.

A sincere thank you to everyone who bought copies of the first printing and conveyed their ideas to me of how to make the book more useful and appealing. I truly appreciated all the feedback and constructive criticism that I received from those who went out of their way to tell me and have included their suggestions in this second edition.

I also want to thank everyone I have had the privilege of working with to help reach their fitness goals. Every person I have worked with has taught me something new about instructing and communicating exercise technique. More than a thousand individuals with their personalities, requirements, interpretations, goals and motivation levels have contributed to bringing this handbook to fruition.

To everyone, I thank you sincerely for your help, support and feedback.

PREFACE

     Weight Training for a New Body is the second edition to my first book, the Weight Trainer's Exercise Handbook. Updated not only with 60 new weight training exercises, you can now easily learn how to develop your own weight training routine to match your fitness goals. In addition, I have also included information on how to perform various stretches to help improve flexibility. The exercises are a compilation of every weight training exercise I have used both in helping people get fit and in my own training as well. The sections on designing your own exercise routine and stretching are as succinct and to-the-point as possible. These sections are designed so that the reader can get started quickly without having to first read half the book. I have also provided many sample exercise routines that I have personally used myself and know that they work well.

     This book was developed to help weight trainers, both novice and those with experience, design their own weight training routine and learn how to perform new exercises properly. It is a reference guide for both exercise prescription and performance. Each exercise is combined with two photographs per page and a written description of each exercise in a consistent format to make learning as easy as possible. The book goes even further than other standard exercise books as it also includes a difficulty rating as well as a starting weight for each exercise.

     Why a starting weight? Is not everybody at a different strength level? It is true that people have different strength levels. However, over the years that I have had the pleasure of working individually with people, I have noticed that most beginner weight trainers start with similar weights. Of course there is variation, but this is not as great as many people would think. Therefore, the weights I have given are only rough approximations for what men and women may consider starting with. Not only do people want to know how to lift weights, they want to know how much weight they should be lifting as well. I hope that these details will make a big difference in the benefits people derive from using this book.

     There can be much discussion over proper exercise technique and appropriateness for any given exercise routine or exercise. Should the elbows be held high? Should you lean into the exercise more? Is too much stress placed on the shoulders or knees? Should I do more sets and fewer repetitions? Should I train this muscle group once or twice a week? Certain exercises are not good for individuals with certain injuries or medical conditions. Some people are not sufficiently physically fit to do other exercises or certain specific routines. Some exercises require a greater degree of flexibility than others do. Would a completely different routine work better or worse? It is essential that those who have doubts or concerns about exercising with weights get the proper instruction for their own unique situation and fitness level. I have done my best, based on my education and experience, to provide you with the most efficient method for learning how to perform weight training exercises properly to work the desired muscle or muscle groups and to combine them into a well structured fitness routine. I hope you find this book both helpful and informative on your quest to better fitness.

INTRODUCTION
HOW TO USE THIS BOOK

This handbook is not designed to be read from cover to cover. It is a reference book to help you develop a weight training routine, find new weight training exercises and to help you learn how to do those exercises properly. The layout is set up to help you learn about weight training routine structuring and the appropriate exercises in as concise a method as possible.

The section on designing a training routine is written to be as brief as possible while still providing all the necessary information to create an exercise program to match your goals. Information on how to choose and place appropriate exercises in your workout, warming up, rest periods, sets, repetitions, how much weight to lift, and how to schedule your workout give you the basic fundamentals on creating a routine. The sections on training for general fitness, muscle definition, muscle development, strength or power give you more specific information and sample routines so that you can create your own customized routine.

How and when to stretch are important in preserving your flexibility. The stretching section contains information on both these topics along with 26 stretches that you can perform to help keep your full range of motion in your joints.

The heart of this book is the exercises. All exercises are grouped together by the main muscle groups that the exercises work. For example, if you wish to find an exercise that works the chest muscles, flip to the *Chest* section and you will find many different chest exercises for strengthening the chest muscles. If you wish to find a specific exercise, there is an index located at the back of the book to help you. In order to help simplify the explanation process there are two pictures for each exercise. Each picture represents the two ranges of motion that you would go through to perform the exercise. It does not represent a full repetition. For example, the dumbbell curl has an illustration showing that the movement starts with the dumbbells on either side of the thighs. The picture labelled "finish" shows the dumbbells held up and in front of the shoulders. This would be as high as you would raise the dumbbells. To do the full repetition you would bring the dumbbells back to the starting position.

You will also notice in the lower right hand corner of the page, under the pictures, a shaded box that looks like this:

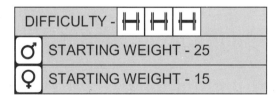

This difficulty rating tells you, on a scale from one to five (illustrated by dumbbells), how difficult the exercise is to learn for the first time. Although learning rate varies from person to person this rating will give you insight into choosing the appropriate exercise for your experience level.

One to two dumbbells – Fairly easy to learn, good exercise for beginners.

Three dumbbells – Somewhat difficult, has some unique movements associated with the exercise that beginners may find awkward.

Four to five dumbbells – This can be a difficult exercise to master. Most beginners will find this awkward but it can be challenging even for advanced lifters.

♂ - represents male starting weight in pounds

 - represents female starting weight in pounds

All starting weights are approximate weights for beginning weight trainers for a repetition range of ten to twelve repetitions per set. The following categories give you additional information on muscle use and detailed descriptions on the execution of the exercises.

MAJOR MUSCLES IN USE: This section signifies which muscle groups (shown in the *Anatomy* section) are being used while performing that particular exercise. In most cases, only the surface muscles that are doing the majority of the work in lifting the weight are outlined here.

STARTING POSITION: Describes the best position to begin the exercise.

EXERCISE MOVEMENT: Describes the motion of the exercise from start to finish.

EXERCISE TECHNIQUE POINTS: Provides tips and pointers for solutions to common problems in performing that particular exercise. Additional notes help you to get the most from the exercise by positioning your body in the optimal position.

INTRODUCTION

Free Weight and Exercise Equipment

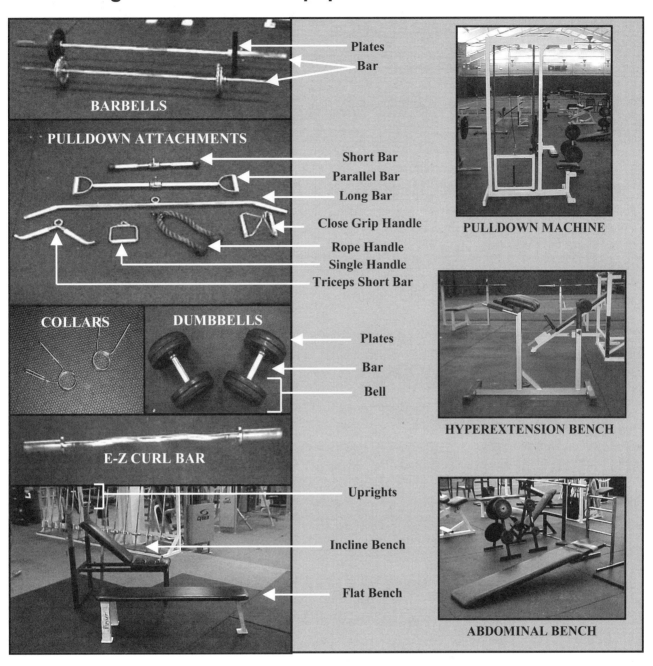

Plates
Bar

BARBELLS

PULLDOWN ATTACHMENTS

Short Bar
Parallel Bar
Long Bar
Close Grip Handle
Rope Handle
Single Handle
Triceps Short Bar

PULLDOWN MACHINE

COLLARS

DUMBBELLS

Plates

Bar

Bell

HYPEREXTENSION BENCH

E-Z CURL BAR

Uprights

Incline Bench

Flat Bench

ABDOMINAL BENCH

Hand Positions

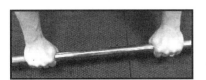

OVERHAND

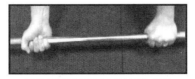

**OVER-UNDERHAND OR
ALTERNATE GRIP**

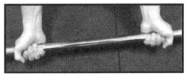

UNDERHAND

TERMINOLOGY

Body Positions

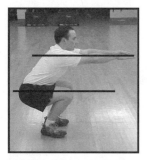

PARALLEL

- Arms and thighs are parallel to the floor.

- Lines on picture are parallel to each other.

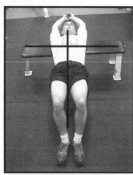

PERPENDICULAR

- Body is perpendicular to the bench.

- Lines represent angle between bench and body.

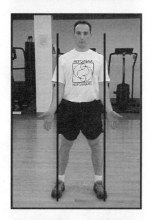

SHOULDER WIDTH

- Feet are shoulder width apart.

- Hands are wider than shoulder width apart.

- Lines represent shoulder width.

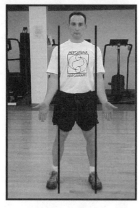

CHEST WIDTH

- Feet are shoulder width apart.

- Lines represent chest width.

TERMINOLOGY

Vocabulary

Repetition - To complete one full movement of the exercise from start to finish. For example, 12 repetitions means lifting the weight twelve times.

Set   - A group of repetitions (for example, 3 sets of 12 repetitions).

Plane   - Along the same axis of movement (for example, along the same path of rotation of the pulley).

Torso   - The upper body.

Trunk   - For the purpose of the book this refers to the midsection involving the abdominal, oblique and lower back muscles.

Spotter   - Someone to assist you in lifting the weight (or performing the exercise) should you find yourself unable to lift or perform the exercise properly on your own.

Work Set - The set of your workout where you are challenging the muscles in order to receive the desired training effect.

Isolation Exercise - This type of exercise tries to focus on one specific muscle group by minimizing the use of other muscles in the movement. An isolation exercise usually involves movement around only one joint.

Compound Exercise - This type of exercise involves several different muscle groups in the movement and involves more than one joint.

DESIGNING AN EXERCISE ROUTINE

Designing a weight training routine can seem like a complicated process. How many sets do I perform? How many repetitions should I do? Should I use 1 or 2 exercises? Which exercises should I choose? How often should I train? Luckily, there are some common training methodologies that can be universally applied to most weight training routines.

EXERCISE SELECTION

The exercises you choose are related to your goals. Obviously, if you wish to have stronger legs you need to choose exercises that involve both the front and rear thigh muscles. Not so obvious is that in order to have strong legs you will also require stronger hips and trunk muscles. Your joints are dependent on many different muscle groups therefore it is always advisable to train all the muscles in the body. This will help to prevent you from developing muscle imbalances and weak areas that may predispose you to injury. If you are training for a particular sport or performance, pick exercises that are close to the movements that you will be doing. For example, squats can help a basketball player jump higher.

It is generally a good idea to choose exercises that involve several different muscle groups or what is referred to as compound exercises. This can make the workout more efficient as you are stressing more than one muscle group at a time. If you wish to specialize on a certain muscle group, choosing isolation exercises (see the definition in the VOCABULARY section) will reduce the involvement of extra muscles. To select an isolation exercise contained in this book, compare the number of muscles used (described under the 'MAJOR MUSCLES IN USE' heading for that movement) between other exercises for the same muscle group and choose the one with the least number of muscles. To pick a compound exercise, choose an exercise that has many muscles listed under the 'MAJOR MUSCLES IN USE' heading.

EXERCISE PLACEMENT

Several factors govern exercise placement when adding exercises to a weight training routine. Muscle groups that play a specific role towards the training goal should be placed before other muscle groups. For example, if you desire a more muscular chest, you should put your chest exercises before other muscle groups. Exercises that involve more muscle mass (compound or multi-joint exercises) should be placed before single joint or isolation exercises. If you are not emphasizing a certain area or do not have a particular goal, muscle groups should be trained from largest to smallest (for example, back should be trained before biceps).

WARM-UP

There are two schools of thought on warming up for weight training. One is to perform some light cardiovascular exercise such as brisk walking, stair climbing, or bike riding for 5 – 10 minutes. This type of exercise helps you to mentally prepare for the workout, increase overall blood flow to the muscles and joints and to help prepare the necessary muscle enzymes for exercise. Another way to warm-up for your weight training workout is to perform warm-up sets. Warm-up sets help to prepare your body and your nervous system for the exercise that it is about to do. Perform 1 - 2 warm-up sets of 5 - 7 repetitions before you begin the work sets for that particular exercise. The weight that you should use for this is approximately 50%-75% of the weight you will use for your work set.

RECOVERY BETWEEN SETS

You should rest approximately 2-3 minutes between sets for the same exercise. This allows the muscle's energy source to regenerate approximately 85% – 95% of pre-exercise levels. If you find that this takes too much time, you may move on to perform another exercise for a different muscle group and then return to the previous exercise. If you choose to do this style of training, make sure you have at least a 2 – 3 minute rest between the same exercise. You may also perform several different exercises in a row. This type of training is referred to as circuit training and is a fast and convenient method for those training for general fitness or to improve stamina. If you are training for muscle development or strength it is advisable to finish all the same sets of the same exercise before moving on to the next.

INTENSITY

You should put a high amount of effort into performing your sets. The weight you choose should be heavy enough so that the last repetition should be difficult to perform. Hard enough that you could maybe get one more of your scheduled repetitions, but definitely no more. However, remember that the last repetition should still be performed in proper form. If you have to "cheat" by not following proper form for your last couple of repetitions, then the weight is too heavy.

REPETITION SELECTION

The number of repetitions you choose for your workout has an effect on how your muscles will respond to the training program you design. Repetition ranges that are above 20 per set causes an increase in muscle tone or firmness of the muscle. You should also notice an increase in the muscle's stamina or endurance. A repetition range of 16 – 20 results in a moderate increase in strength, a slight increase in muscle development as well as an increase in stamina. Choosing repetitions from 12 – 15 causes a greater increase in strength and muscle development and less of a stamina or endurance effect. A repetition range of 8 – 11 is optimal for muscle development and good for increasing strength. One would also see an increase in muscle tone but only a slight increase in muscle stamina. For those whose sole goal is to increase strength, a repetition range from 4 – 7 results in optimal strength gain, good muscle development, good muscle tone but poor muscle endurance. Ultimately, the number of repetitions you choose depends on your fitness goals and level of experience. For more detail on these factors, consult the sections within this chapter on training for specific goals.

SCHEDULING YOUR WORKOUT

The best schedule that you can choose is one that gives you the most consistency in your workouts. For example, would your rather exercise 3 times a week for an hour each time or 5 times a week for 30 minutes? Which days can you not exercise? What time of day could you set aside some time to yourself? Do you need a workout schedule with some flexibility? All these factors control your schedule and ultimately how successful you will be in achieving your goal. Depending on the reason for which you are exercising, your muscles require a certain number of sets and repetitions in order to improve. This is outlined in the following sections on training for specific goals. Based on this information you can construct different routines to match your schedule.

There is some flexibility as to when you can train certain muscle groups since your muscles require time to recover and adapt to the workout. How much time they require depends on the set and repetition ranges. There is more detailed information on this topic in the following sections. Training different muscle groups on different days is the most common way of designing a routine to fit various schedules. You may decide to split your muscle groups up over 2, 3, 4 or even more days depending on your goals. The following splits give some examples of how you can divide up your muscle groups over several days.

DESIGNING AN EXERCISE ROUTINE   7

2 Day Split Version A

Day 1 – Back, Chest, Shoulders, Abdominals
Day 2 – Front Thigh, Rear Thigh, Biceps,
          Triceps, Calves

2 Day Split Version B

Day 1 – Shoulders, Biceps, Triceps,
          Abdominals, Calves
Day 2 – Front Thigh, Rear Thigh, Back, Chest

2 Day Split Version C

Day 1 – Chest, Biceps, Triceps, Front Thigh,
          Calves
Day 2 – Back, Shoulders, Rear Thigh,
          Abdominals

2 Day Split Version D

Day 1 – Back, Biceps, Rear Thigh,
          Abdominals
Day 2 – Chest, Triceps, Front Thigh,
          Shoulders

3 Day Split Version A

Day 1 – Back, Shoulders, Abdominals
Day 2 – Front Thigh, Rear Thigh, Calves
Day 3 – Chest, Biceps, Triceps

3 Day Split Version B

Day 1 – Back, Biceps, Abdominals
Day 2 – Front Thigh, Rear Thigh, Shoulders
Day 3 – Chest, Triceps, Calves

3 Day Split Version C

Day 1 – Chest, Back, Abdominals
Day 2 – Front Thigh, Rear Thigh, Calves
Day 3 – Shoulders, Biceps, Triceps

3 Day Split Version D

Day 1 – Shoulders, Abdominals, Calves
Day 2 – Front Thigh, Back, Triceps
Day 3 – Rear Thigh, Chest, Biceps

4 Day Split Version A

Day 1 – Back, Abdominals
Day 2 – Front Thigh, Rear Thigh
Day 3 – Chest, Biceps, Triceps
Day 4 - Shoulders, Calves

4 Day Split Version B

Day 1 – Chest, Triceps
Day 2 – Front Thigh, Calves
Day 3 – Shoulders, Rear Thigh
Day 4 – Back, Biceps, Abdominals

4 Day Split Version C

Day 1 – Biceps, Rear Thighs, Abdominals
Day 2 – Calves, Shoulders
Day 3 – Triceps, Front Thighs
Day 4 - Back, Chest

4 Day Split Version D

Day 1 – Rear Thigh, Triceps
Day 2 – Front Thigh, Biceps
Day 3 – Back, Shoulders
Day 4 – Chest, Abdominals, Calves

5 Day Split Version A

Day 1 – Back, Abdominals
Day 2 – Chest, Calves
Day 3 – Shoulders, Forearms
Day 4 – Biceps, Triceps
Day 5 – Front Thigh, Rear Thigh

5 Day Split Version B

Day 1 – Biceps, Front Thigh
Day 2 – Triceps, Rear Thigh
Day 3 – Chest, Abdominals
Day 4 – Back, Calves
Day 5 – Shoulders

DESIGNING AN EXERCISE ROUTINE

TRAINING FOR GENERAL FITNESS

What kind of results can I expect from training for general fitness?

People who train for general fitness with weights have a wide variety of goals and are looking for improvement in all the major areas including fat loss, strength, muscle definition and muscle development. One disadvantage to having such a broad approach is that progress is not as rapid in all the areas than if just one specific goal was chosen such as increasing muscle development.

How many sets and repetitions should I do for each muscle group?

The total number of sets and repetitions that you choose for each muscle group depends on your level of experience. The more experienced a lifter, the more sets and varied repetitions the muscles can tolerate. The table below gives a guideline based on experience level.

Goal	Experience	Repetitions	Sets	Estimated Rest Days
General Fitness	None	15 -20	1 – 2	2 - 3
	2 weeks	15	2 – 3	3
	6 – 8 weeks	12 - 15	3 – 4	3
	6 months	10 – 15	4	3 - 4
	> 12 months	8 - 20	5 - 6	4

The total number of sets for individuals with no experience begins with 1 – 2 sets per muscle group. If you find that your muscles are not very sore a few days after completing the workout, you may add 1 set to the total number of sets before the 2-week period. As the table outlines, you can continue to add 1 set for each muscle group every several months. However, it is possible you can still get results from staying in the 3 - 4 set range for years.

Repetitions are set in the range of 15 - 20 for beginners. This is to reduce the risk of injury in the first few weeks from lifting weights that may be too heavy for the muscles and tendons. As your muscles adapt to the training, you may wish to decrease the repetitions to help increase strength and muscle development.

Estimated Rest Days can also vary with experience level but are closely associated with the number of sets you perform in your workout. Even though the longer you train, your body learns to increase its recovery ability, you can also push yourself harder and tolerate a more strenuous workout. This results in a required rest period that is longer between workouts the more experienced you become.

SAMPLE GENERAL FITNESS ROUTINES

Whole Body Weight Training Schedule for 2 - 3 times a Week

Example Workout Schedule for 2 times a week:

SUN.	MON.	TUES.	WED.	THURS.	FRI.	SAT.
Rest	Weight Training	Rest	Rest	Weight Training	Rest	Rest

Example Workout Schedule for 3 times a week:

SUN.	MON.	TUES.	WED.	THURS.	FRI.	SAT.
Rest	Weight Training	Rest	Weight Training	Rest	Weight Training	Rest

Beginner General Fitness Sample Routine

Exercises	Sets	Reps
Bent Over Dumbbell Row	2 - 3	15
Flat Dumbbell Fly	2 – 3	15
Side Laterals	2 – 3	15
Kickbacks	2 – 3	15
Floor Twist Crunches	2 – 3	15
Concentration Curls	2 – 3	15
Split Squats	2 – 3	15
Stiff Leg Deadlift	2 – 3	15
Calf Raises	2 - 3	15

Alternate Beginner General Fitness Sample Routine

Exercises	Sets	Reps
Wide Grip Lat Pulldown to the Front	2 – 3	15
Flat Dumbbell Fly	2 – 3	15
Upright Row	2 – 3	15
Triceps Pushdowns	2 – 3	15
Dumbbell Curls	2 – 3	15
Leg Press	2 – 3	15
Prone Leg Curls	2 – 3	15
Incline Leg Raise	2 – 3	15
Seated Calf Raises	2 - 3	15

2 Day Split Weight Training Schedule for 3 or 4 times a week

Example Workout Schedule for 3 times a week:

WEEK	SUN.	MON.	TUES.	WED.	THURS.	FRI.	SAT.
1	Rest	Day 1	Rest	Day 2	Rest	Day 1	Rest
2	Rest	Day 2	Rest	Day 1	Rest	Day 2	Rest

Example Workout Schedule for 4 times a week:

SUN.	MON.	TUES.	WED.	THURS.	FRI.	SAT.
Rest	Day 1	Day 2	Rest	Day 1	Day 2	Rest

Muscle	Day 1 Exercises	Sets	Reps
Back	Reverse Grip Pulldown	2 - 3	15
Back	Seated Row	2	15
Chest	Bench Press	2 -3	15
Chest	Incline Flyes	2	15
Shoulders	Side Laterals	3	15
Abdominal	Hanging Leg Raises	3	15

Muscle	Day 2 Exercises	Sets	Reps
Triceps	Triceps Pushdown	3	15
Biceps	Dumbbell Curls	3	15
Thigh and Hip	Squats	3	15
Rear Thigh	Stiff Leg Deadlift	3	15
Abdominal	Ball Crunches	3	15
Calf	Single Leg Calf Raise	3	15

3 Day Split Advanced Weight Training Schedule for 5 - 6 times a week

WEEK	SUN.	MON.	TUES.	WED.	THURS.	FRI.	SAT.
1	Day 1	Day 2	Day 3	Rest	Day 1	Day 2	Day 3
2	Rest	Day 1	Day 2	Day 3	Rest	Day 1	Day 2
3	Day 3	Rest	Day 1	Day 2	Day 3	Rest	Day 1
4	Day 2	Day 3	Rest	Day 1	Day 2	Day 3	Rest

Muscle	Day 1 Exercises	Sets	Reps
Chest	Incline Barbell Press	3	12
Chest	Cable Cross-Overs	3	12
Back	Close Grip Pulldowns	3	12
Back	Bent Over Row	3	12
Abdominal	Cable Crunch	3	15
Abdominal	Bicycle Crunch	3	15

Muscle	Day 2 Exercises	Sets	Reps
Thigh and Hip	One Legged Press	3	12
Quadriceps	Leg Extension	3	12
Hamstrings	Ball Leg Curl	3	12
Rear Thigh	Seated Leg Curl	3	12
Calf	Calf Raises	3	15
Calf	Single Leg Calf Raise	3	15

Muscle	Day 3 Exercises	Sets	Reps
Front Shoulder	Seated Dumbbell Shoulder Press	2	12
Side Shoulder	Cable Side Laterals	3	12
Rear Shoulder	Bent Over Laterals	2	12
Biceps	Body Drag Curl	4	12
Triceps	Standing Cable Triceps Extension	4	12

TRAINING FOR MUSCLE DEFINITION

What kind of results can I expect from training for muscle definition?

Weight training to increase muscle definition is currently one of the most popular training goals. To have good muscle definition means to be able to clearly see the shape of each muscle on your body. In some cases, you may even notice the bundles of muscle fibres that give the muscle an almost corded appearance when tensed. Good muscle definition occurs when there is a combination of having minimal amounts of body fat over well-developed muscles. The degree of muscle development can be tailored to the individual's taste, however it is important to remember that small muscles do not look as defined as more developed muscles. Training for muscle definition incorporates using a higher number of repetitions and sets to help increase the total amount of calories burned. This approach helps to decrease body fat while working towards building some muscle.

How many sets and repetitions should I do for each muscle group?

The total number of sets and repetitions that you choose for each muscle group depends on your level of experience. The more experienced a lifter you are, the more sets and varied repetitions your muscles can tolerate. The table below gives a guideline based on experience level.

Goal	Experience	Repetitions	Sets	Estimated Rest Days
Muscle Definition	None	20	3	2 - 3
	2 months	15	4	3
	4 months	15	5	4
	6 months	12 – 15	6	4
	> 12 months	15	8 - 12	5 - 6

Total number of sets for individuals with no experience begins with 3 sets per muscle group. If you find that your muscles are not too sore a few days after completing the workout, you may add 1 set to the total number of sets before the 2-week period. You can continue to add 1 set for each muscle group every several months as the table outlines.

Repetitions are set in the range of 20 for beginners. This is to reduce the risk of injury in the first few weeks from lifting weights that may be too heavy for the muscles and tendons. In addition, the higher number of repetitions also causes more calories to be burned resulting in a faster reduction of body fat levels. As your body becomes trained over the months, you may decrease the repetitions and increase the number of sets to help stimulate some muscle development. As your body builds muscle, its overall metabolism increases resulting in more calories being burned at rest and while exercising. You should notice more definition and improved shape as your muscles develop.

How much body fat your body loses is ultimately determined by how great of a caloric deficit (calories consumed from food minus calories used for life functions, daily activities and exercise) you create in your body. Following a nutritionally balanced and lower calorie diet is essential to your success in achieving your goal. I would recommend speaking to your family physician or a registered dietician if you require specific information on this topic.

Estimated Rest Days can also vary with experience level but are closely associated with the number of sets you perform in your workout. The longer you train, your body learns to increase its recovery ability. From this adaptation you can push yourself harder and tolerate a more challenging workout.

SAMPLE MUSCLE DEFINITION ROUTINES

Whole Body Weight Training Schedule for 2 or 3 times a week

Example Workout Schedule for 2 times a week:

SUN.	MON.	TUES.	WED.	THURS.	FRI.	SAT.
Rest	Weight Training	Rest	Rest	Weight Training	Rest	Rest

Example Workout Schedule for 3 times a week:

SUN.	MON.	TUES.	WED.	THURS.	FRI.	SAT.
Rest	Weight Training	Rest	Weight Training	Rest	Weight Training	Rest

Beginner Sample Muscle Definition Routine

Muscle	Day 1 Exercises	Sets	Reps
Back	One Arm Row	3	20
Chest	Incline Dumbbell Fly	3	20
Shoulders	Side Laterals	3	20
Triceps	Kickbacks	3	20
Abdominal	Incline Twist Crunches	3	20
Biceps	Concentration Curls	3	20
Thigh and Hip	Walking Lunges	3	20
Rear Thigh	Stiff Leg Deadlift	3	20
Calf	Calf Raises	3	20

Alternate Beginner Sample Muscle Definition Routine

Muscle	Day 1 Exercises	Sets	Reps
Back	Wide Grip Lat Pulldown to the Front	3	20
Chest	Flat Dumbbell Fly	3	20
Shoulders	Upright Row	3	20
Triceps	Triceps Pushdowns	3	20
Biceps	Dumbbell Curls	3	20
Thigh and Hip	Leg Press	3	20
Rear Thigh	Prone Leg Curls	3	20
Abdominal	Incline Leg Raise	3	20
Calf	Seated Calf Raises	3	20

2 Day Split Weight Training Schedule for 3 or 4 times a week

Example Workout Schedule for 3 times a week:

WEEK	SUN.	MON.	TUES.	WED.	THURS.	FRI.	SAT.
1	Rest	Day 1	Rest	Day 2	Rest	Day 1	Rest
2	Rest	Day 2	Rest	Day 1	Rest	Day 2	Rest

Example Workout Schedule for 4 times a week:

SUN.	MON.	TUES.	WED.	THURS.	FRI.	SAT.
Rest	Day 1	Day 2	Rest	Day 1	Day 2	Rest

Muscle	Day 1 Exercises	Sets	Reps
Back	One Arm Lat Pulldown	3	15
Back	Cable Stiff Arm Pullover	3	15
Chest	Incline Dumbbell Press	3	15
Chest	Decline Dumbbell Flyes	3	15
Shoulders	Cable Upright Row	3	15
Rear Shoulders	One Arm Bent Over Laterals	3	15
Abdominal	Hanging Leg Raises	3	15

Muscle	Day 2 Exercises	Sets	Reps
Triceps	Triceps Pushdown	3	15
Triceps	Seated Triceps Ext.	3	15
Biceps	Barbell Curls	3	15
Biceps	Incline Curls	3	15
Front Thigh	Leg Extension	3	15
Thigh and Hip	Reverse Lunges	3	15
Rear Thigh	Cable Leg Curl	3	15
Buttocks	Straight Leg Kickback	2	15

4 Day Split Advanced Weight Training Schedule for 5 - 6 times a week

WEEK	SUN.	MON.	TUES.	WED.	THURS.	FRI.	SAT.
1	Day 1	Day 2	Day 3	Day 4	Rest	Day 1	Day 2
2	Day 3	Day 4	Rest	Day 1	Day 2	Day 3	Day 4
3	Rest	Day 1	Day 2	Day 3	Day 4	Rest	Day 1
4	Day 2	Day 3	Day 4	Rest	Day 1	Day 2	Day 3
5	Day 4	Rest	Day 1	Day 2	Day 3	Day 4	Rest

Muscle	Day 1 Exercises	Sets	Reps
Chest	Incline Press	4	12
Thigh and Hip	One Legged Squat	4	12
Chest	Flat Dumbbell Press	4	12
Front Thigh	Bar Hack Squat	4	12
Chest	Bench Press	4	12
Thigh and Hip	Lunges	4	12

Muscle	Day 2 Exercises	Sets	Reps
Front Shoulders	Arnold Press	4	12
Abdominals	Full Incline Crunch	4	15
Side Shoulders	Seated Side Laterals	4	12
Obliques	Side Crunch	4	15
Rear Shoulder	Bent Over Laterals	4	12
Abdominals	V's	4	15

Muscle	Day 3 Exercises	Sets	Reps
Back	Single Arm Pullover	4	12
Triceps	Close Grip Press	4	12
Back	Reverse Grip Bent Over Row	4	12
Triceps	Cross Bench Triceps Ext.	4	12
Back	Lat Pulldowns to the Rear	4	12
Triceps	Incline Lying Tricep Extension	4	12

Muscle	Day 4 Exercises	Sets	Reps
Biceps	Alternate Dumbbell Curl	4	12
Rear Thigh	Stiff Leg Deadlifts	4	12
Biceps	Hammer Curls	4	12
Rear Thigh	Prone Leg Curls	4	12
Biceps	Spider Curls	4	12
Rear Thigh	Single Leg Curls	4	12

TRAINING FOR MUSCLE DEVELOPMENT

What kind of results can I expect from training for muscle development?

If you are training for muscle development your main goal is to increase the size of your muscles. As a secondary goal you may also desire greater strength and muscle definition. This results as a by-product of the muscle increasing in size. Muscle size can be correlated to the strength of the muscle, while a larger muscle appears more defined because you can see it better.

How many sets and repetitions should I do for each muscle group?

The total number of sets and repetitions that you choose for each muscle group depends on your level of experience. The more experienced weight trainer you are, the wider variety of training you can do. The table below gives a guideline based on experience level.

Goal	Experience	Repetitions	Sets	Estimated Rest Days
Muscle Development	None	15	3	2 - 3
	1 month	12	3	3 - 4
	3 months	10	5	4 – 5
	6 months	8	6	5 – 6
	10 months	10 - 12	8 - 12	6 - 8
	At 12 months repeat from 1 month but reduce repetitions to 10 per set.			

The total number of sets that beginners should start with is 3 sets per muscle. If you find that your muscles are very sore a few days after completing the workout, you may decrease the total number of sets by 1 set before the first month is over. As the table outlines, you can continue to increase the number of sets for each muscle group every several months. Unlike training for general fitness, it is necessary to vary the number of sets per muscle group to optimize muscle growth. At about the year mark where you have completed at least 12 sets for each body part, it is necessary to drastically reduce your number of sets to continue to increase muscle size at an optimal rate. It is also advisable to train for strength at least once a year in order to ensure that your nervous system is operating at a high level to properly activate your muscles.

Repetitions are set in the range of 15 for beginners. This is to reduce the risk of injury in the first few weeks from lifting weights that may be too heavy for the muscles and tendons. As the muscles adapt to the training, you should slowly decrease the number of repetitions every few months to continue to stimulate the muscle to develop.

Estimated Rest Days can also vary with experience level but are closely associated with the number of sets you perform in your workout. The ranges shown act as a guideline and can vary with age, nutrition, and activity patterns. If you find that the weights you are lifting are not increasing every 2 – 3 weeks or that you have consistently sore muscles, choose the higher number in the range. It is almost always better to have slightly more rest than to not have enough.

SAMPLE MUSCLE DEVELOPMENT ROUTINES

Example Workout Schedule for 2 times a week:

SUN.	MON.	TUES.	WED.	THURS.	FRI.	SAT.
Rest	Weight Training	Rest	Rest	Weight Training	Rest	Rest

Example Workout Schedule for 3 times a week:

SUN.	MON.	TUES.	WED.	THURS.	FRI.	SAT.
Rest	Weight Training	Rest	Weight Training	Rest	Weight Training	Rest

Beginner Sample Muscle Development Routine

Muscle	Day 1 Exercises	Sets	Reps
Back	Bent Over Row	3	12
Chest	Bench Press	3	12
Shoulders	Upright Row	3	12
Triceps	Lying Barbell Triceps Extension	3	12
Biceps	Barbell Curls	3	12
Abdominal	Incline Crunch	3	12
Thigh and Hip	Squats	3	12
Rear Thigh	Stiff Leg Deadlift	3	12
Calf	Calf Raises	3	12

Alternate Beginner Sample Muscle Definition Routine

Muscle	Day 1 Exercises	Sets	Reps
Back	Reverse Grip Pulldown	3	12
Chest	Flat Dumbbell Press	3	12
Shoulders	Upright Row	3	12
Triceps	Triceps Pushdowns	3	12
Biceps	Dumbbell Curls	3	12
Thigh and Hip	Leg Press	3	12
Rear Thigh	Prone Leg Curls	3	12
Abdominal	Incline Leg Raise	3	20
Calf	Seated Calf Raises	3	20

2 Day Split Weight Training Schedule for 3 or 4 times a week

Example Workout Schedule for 3 times a week:

WEEK	SUN.	MON.	TUES.	WED.	THURS.	FRI.	SAT.
1	Rest	Day 1	Rest	Day 2	Rest	Day 1	Rest
2	Rest	Day 2	Rest	Day 1	Rest	Day 2	Rest

Example Workout Schedule for 4 times a week:

SUN.	MON.	TUES.	WED.	THURS.	FRI.	SAT.
Rest	Day 1	Day 2	Rest	Day 1	Day 2	Rest

Muscle	Day 1 Exercises	Sets	Reps
Chest	Flat Dumbbell Press	2	10
Chest	Incline Flyes	2	10
Back	Wide Grip Pulldown	3	10
Back	T-Bar Row	2	10
Shoulders	Side Laterals	3	10
Rear Shoulders	Standing One Arm Cable Rear Laterals	2	10
Abdominal	Hanging Leg Raises	3	15

Muscle	Day 2 Exercises	Sets	Reps
Thigh and Hip	Split Squats	3	10
Front Thigh	One Legged Ext.	2	10
Rear Thigh	Stiff Leg Deadlift	2	10
Rear Thigh	One Legged Curl	2	10
Biceps	Incline Curls	4	10
Triceps	Seated Triceps Ext.	4	10
Calf	Toe Presses	3	12

3 Day Split Advanced Weight Training Schedule for 5 - 6 times a week

WEEK	SUN.	MON.	TUES.	WED.	THURS.	FRI.	SAT.
1	Day 1	Day 2	Day 3	Rest	Day 1	Day 2	Day 3
2	Rest	Day 1	Day 2	Day 3	Rest	Day 1	Day 2
3	Day 3	Rest	Day 1	Day 2	Day 3	Rest	Day 1
4	Day 2	Day 3	Rest	Day 1	Day 2	Day 3	Rest

Muscle	Day 1 Exercises	Sets	Reps
Chest	Incline Dumbbell Press	3	8
Chest	Flat Flyes	3	8
Biceps	Preacher Curl	3	10
Biceps	Incline Curls	2	10
Triceps	Lying Triceps Ext.	3	10
Triceps	Seated French Press	2	10

Muscle	Day 2 Exercises	Sets	Reps
Thigh and Hip	Squats	3	8
Quadriceps	Leg Extension	3	8
Rear Thigh	Stiff Leg Deadlift	3	8
Rear Thigh	Prone Leg Curl	3	8
Calves	Standing Calf Raise	3	12
Abdominals	Weighted Incline Twist Crunch	3	12

Muscle	Day 3 Exercises	Sets	Reps
Back	Wide Grip Pulldown	3	8
Back	Seated Row	3	8
Front Shoulders	Military Press	2	8
Side Shoulder	Side Laterals	2	10
Rear Shoulder	Bent Over Laterals	2	10
Abdominals	Hanging Leg Raise	3	12

DESIGNING AN EXERCISE ROUTINE 18

TRAINING FOR STRENGTH

What kind of results can I expect from training for strength?

If you are training for strength your number one priority is to increase the strength of your muscles. There are several different definitions of strength. For the purpose of this book, strength is defined as the maximum amount of weight you can lift once. There is also a good correlation between maximum strength and the number of times you can lift a lighter weight. For example, currently you can lift 20 pounds above your head 15 times. After training for strength you can now lift that 20 pounds 25 times above your head. When training for strength you may notice other improvements in muscle development and muscle tone.

How many sets and repetitions should I do for each muscle group?

The total number of sets and repetitions that you choose for each muscle group depends on your level of experience. The more experienced weight trainer you become, the more intensely you can train and the heavier a weight you can lift. The table below gives a guideline based on experience level.

Goal	Experience	Repetitions	Sets	Estimated Rest Days
Strength	None	15	3	3
	3 months	10	4	3 - 4
	6 months	8	5	4 – 5
	> 1 year	3 – 6	6	5 – 6

The total number of sets begins with 3 sets per muscle group for those who have no experience lifting weights. If you find that your muscles are very sore a few days after completing the workout, you may decrease 1 set from the total number of sets before you reach the third month. As the table outlines, you can continue to increase the number of sets for each muscle group every several months. Unlike training for muscle development, it is not necessary to perform a high number of sets. In fact, it is usually counter-productive to perform more than 6 sets for each muscle group even after you have been training for several years. It is important to note that muscle strength is also related to the size of your muscles. Therefore, at some point in your training it is wise to train for muscle development for 3 – 6 months.

Repetitions are set in the range of 15 for beginners. This is to reduce the risk of injury in the first few weeks from lifting weights that may be too heavy for the muscles and tendons. As the muscles adapt to the training, you should slowly decrease the number of repetitions every few months to continue to stimulate the muscle and nervous system to become stronger.

Estimated Rest Days can also vary with experience level but are closely associated with the number of sets you perform in your workout. The ranges are merely guidelines and can vary with age, nutrition, and activity patterns. If you find that the weights you are lifting are not increasing every 2 – 3 weeks or that you have consistently sore muscles, choose the higher number of rest days in the range. It is almost always better to have slightly more rest than to not have enough.

SAMPLE STRENGTH TRAINING ROUTINES

Example Workout Schedule for 2 times a week:

SUN.	MON.	TUES.	WED.	THURS.	FRI.	SAT.
Rest	Weight Training	Rest	Rest	Weight Training	Rest	Rest

Example Workout Schedule for 3 times a week:

SUN.	MON.	TUES.	WED.	THURS.	FRI.	SAT.
Rest	Weight Training	Rest	Weight Training	Rest	Weight Training	Rest

Beginner Sample Strength Routine

Muscle	Day 1 Exercises	Sets	Reps
Back	Bent Over Row	3	12
Chest	Bench Press	3	12
Shoulders	Upright Row	3	12
Triceps	Lying Barbell Triceps Extension	3	12
Biceps	Barbell Curls	3	12
Abdominal	Incline Crunch	3	12
Thigh and Hip	Squats	3	12
Rear Thigh	Stiff Leg Deadlift	3	12
Calf	Calf Raises	3	12

Alternate Beginner Sample Strength Routine

Muscle	Day 1 Exercises	Sets	Reps
Back	Reverse Grip Pulldown	3	12
Chest	Flat Dumbbell Press	3	12
Shoulders	Upright Row	3	12
Triceps	Triceps Pushdowns	3	12
Biceps	Dumbbell Curls	3	12
Thigh and Hip	Leg Press	3	12
Rear Thigh	Prone Leg Curls	3	12
Abdominal	Incline Leg Raise	3	20
Calf	Seated Calf Raises	3	20

2 Day Split Weight Training Schedule for 3 - 4 times a week

2 Day Split Weight Training Schedule for 3 times a week:

WEEK	SUN.	MON.	TUES.	WED.	THURS.	FRI.	SAT.
1	Rest	Day 1	Rest	Day 2	Rest	Day 1	Rest
2	Rest	Day 2	Rest	Day 1	Rest	Day 2	Rest

2 Day Split Weight Training Schedule for 4 times a week:

SUN.	MON.	TUES.	WED.	THURS.	FRI.	SAT.
Rest	Day 1	Day 2	Rest	Day 1	Day 2	Rest

Muscle	Day 1 Exercises	Sets	Reps
Chest	Flat Dumbbell Press	2	8
Chest	Incline Flyes	2	8
Back	Wide Grip Pulldown	2	8
Back	One Arm Row	2	8
Shoulders	Side Laterals	3	10
Rear Shoulders	Standing One Arm Cable Rear Laterals	2	10
Abdominal	Hanging Leg Raises	3	15

Muscle	Day 2 Exercises	Sets	Reps
Thigh and Hip	Squats	2	8
Front Thigh	Leg Press	2	8
Rear Thigh	Stiff Leg Deadlift	2	8
Rear Thigh	One Legged Curl	2	8
Biceps	Barbell Curls	3	8
Triceps	Narrow Grip Press	3	8
Calf	Toe Presses	3	10

3 Day Split Advanced Weight Training Schedule for 5 - 6 times a week

WEEK	SUN.	MON.	TUES.	WED.	THURS.	FRI.	SAT.
1	Rest	Day 1	Rest	Day 2	Day 3	Rest	Day 1
2	Day 2	Day 3	Rest	Day 1a	Day 2a	Day 3a	Rest

* Exercises are to be performed explosively from the lowered position.

Muscle	Day 1 Exercises	Sets	Reps
Shoulder	Military Press*	3	6,4,3
Shoulder	Upright Row	2	8
Back	Bent Over Row	3	6
Abdominal	Incline Twist Crunch	3	15

Muscle	Day 2 Exercises	Sets	Reps
Chest	Bench Press*	3	6,4,3
Chest	Incline Flyes	1	10
Triceps	Close Grip Bench*	3	6,4,3
Biceps	Arm Curl	3	9

Muscle	Day 3 Exercises	Sets	Reps
Front Thigh and Hip	Squat	3	6,4,3
Calves	Calves	3	9
Lower Body and Back	Deadlift	3	6,4,3
Forearm	Wrist Curl	2	9
Forearm	Wrist Extension	2	9

Muscle	Day 1a Exercises	Sets	Reps
Front Shoulder	Military Press*	3	15
Side Shoulder	Side Lateral Raise	2	9
Back	Wide Grip Pulldown to the Front	3	9
Rear Shoulder	Bent-Over Laterals	2	9
Abdominal	Incl. Twist Crunch*	3	12

Muscle	Day 2a Exercises	Sets	Reps
Chest	Bench Press*	3	15
Chest	Incline Press	1	9
Triceps	Close Grip Press*	3	15
Biceps	Dumbbell Curl	3	9

Muscle	Day 3a Exercises	Sets	Reps
Thigh and Hip	Squat*	3	15
Lower Body and Back	Deadlift*	3	15
Rear Thigh	Leg Curl	2	12
Calves	Calves	3	12
Forearms	Wrist Curl	2	9
Forearms	Wrist Extension	2	9

TRAINING FOR POWER

What kind of results can I expect from training for power?

If you are training for power your goal is to increase the amount of weight you can move quickly. For example, some one who can jump high is said to have powerful legs because they can move their legs quick enough to propel their bodyweight high above the ground. An athlete who can throw a discus farther than another probably has more power than his or her opponent. As you can probably guess, athletes most commonly train for power. Integrating a power routine can be a complicated process and is best left to a fitness professional who is familiar with this type of training. The guidelines outlined in this chapter will give you an introduction as to how you can increase your power. There is also a good correlation between a high strength level and a high power output, however one does not guarantee the other. When training for power you will notice an increase in strength as well as an increase in the speed at which you can lift a heavy weight or move your body. You may notice other slight improvements in muscle development and muscle tone.

How many sets and repetitions should I do for each muscle group?

Power training should only be performed after at least 6 months of consistent strength training and should be developed by a fitness professional or coach who is knowledgeable in power training. The total number of sets and repetitions that you choose for each muscle group depends on your level of experience. The more experienced a weight trainer you become, the more intensely you can train and therefore the heavier a weight you can lift. The table below gives a guideline based on experience level.

Goal	Experience	Repetitions	Sets	Estimated Rest Days
Power (repetitions are performed at an explosive speed)	6 months	5 - 8	3	3
	9 months	4 - 6	4	3 - 4
	12 months	3 – 5	3 – 5	4 – 5
	Elite	1 – 3	6 – 10	5 – 6

Total number of sets begins with 3 sets per muscle group for those who have no experience with power training with weights. If you find that your muscles are very sore a few days after completing the workout, you may decrease 1 set from the total number of sets before the 3 month period is over. As the table outlines, you can continue to increase the number of sets for each muscle group every several months. Similar to strength training, it is necessary to increase your number of sets as you decrease your number of repetitions. Often you can be performing 2 repetitions per set for up to 10 sets at various stages of your training. It is important to remember that muscle power is also related to the strength and size of your muscles. Therefore at some point in your training it is wise to train for muscle development and strength for several months at a time. In addition, training for power involves training at such a high intensity level that you can become over trained quickly if you are not careful.

Repetitions are set in the range of 5 - 8 for those who are new to power training. This is to reduce the risk of injury from lifting weights in an explosive manner. This type of training can place a heavy strain on muscles and tendons and therefore needs a conditioning period to get used to the intensity level. As the muscles adapt to the training, you should slowly decrease the number of repetitions every few months to continue to stimulate the muscle and nervous system to become more powerful.

Estimated Rest Days can also vary with experience level but are closely associated with the number of sets you perform in your workout. The ranges are given as guidelines and can vary with age, nutrition, and activity patterns. If you find that the weights you are lifting are not increasing every 2 – 3 weeks or that you have consistently sore muscles, choose the higher number of rest days in the range. It is almost always better to have slightly more rest than to not have enough.

2 Day Split Weight Training Schedule for 3 or 4 times a week

Example Workout Schedule for 3 times a week:

WEEK	SUN.	MON.	TUES.	WED.	THURS.	FRI.	SAT.
1	Rest	Day 1	Rest	Day 2	Rest	Day 1	Rest
2	Rest	Day 2	Rest	Day 1	Rest	Day 2	Rest

Example Workout Schedule for 4 times a week:

SUN.	MON.	TUES.	WED.	THURS.	FRI.	SAT.
Rest	Day 1	Day 2	Rest	Day 1	Day 2	Rest

* - Exercises are to be performed explosively from the lowered position

Muscle	Day 1 Exercises	Sets	Reps
Chest	Flat Dumbbell Press*	3	8
Thigh and Hip	Squats*	3	8,6,6
Thigh and Hip	Side Lunges*	3	8,6,6
Back	Bent Over Row*	3	8
Lower Body and Back	Deadlift*	3	6
Lower Back	Back Extension	3	15

Muscle	Day 2 Exercises	Sets	Reps
Upper Body	Hang Cleans*	3	6
Front Shoulder	Push Press*	3	6
Triceps	Narrow Grip Press*	3	6
Abdominals	Cable Crunch	3	12
Calf	Smith Machine Calf Raise*	3	8
Obliques	Standing Cable Torso Rotation	3	15
Calf	Toe Presses*	3	10

The above routine was designed as an introduction to power training and is not representative of an advanced power routine. More advanced power routines should be tailored to the individuals goals and be as specific as possible. For more information consult a qualified fitness professional.

PUTTING IT ALL TOGETHER

As you may have realized by now, there are many different ways to create a weight training routine. Most routines will give some results, although a well-structured routine will give you faster and more noticeable progress. Choose an exercise schedule that will fit with your lifestyle. Depending on your goal, try a 2, 3, 4-day split or more to give yourself the necessary recovery time and flexibility in arranging your workout. If you are training with fewer than 6 sets per body part, make sure you exercise each muscle group twice a week. Greater than 6 sets and you may require a week to recover. Train the areas you want to improve the most first in your routine. Rest between sets for the same muscle group for 2 – 3 minutes (you can accomplish this by either waiting or by performing circuit training) and allow at least 72 hours to pass before you train the same area again. Start slow and build up the weight you are using by progressing to less repetitions per set. However, always make sure that the last repetition of your set is difficult to get using proper form. This will cause the stimulus necessary for your muscles to change and get stronger, more defined, well developed, and firm to the touch.

A FINAL NOTE

The application of the various tables for sets, repetitions and sample workouts will vary according to your specific goal and fitness level. It is important to closely monitor your progress and record your workout each time. This allows you to consistently keep track of your performance for each workout and help identify problems that may arise such as over-training. This condition is perhaps one of the most common reasons for lack of progress. Over-training happens when the body can not recover in time from the previous training session before the muscles are trained again. Mild over-training can cause such problems as stalled progress and poor results. Chronic, extreme over-training can result in decreased strength, over-use injuries, a poorly functioning immune system, and hormone changes.   Adequate rest is just as important as training hard. Full recovery times for weight training can be as little 48 hours to a full 14 days before the muscle has recovered and is ready to be trained again. Recovery times can vary due to the effects of volume, intensity, past training experience, sleeping habits, nutrition status, stress levels, and even genetic disposition.

STRETCHING

Flexibility is an important part of any fitness program. Performing stretching exercises helps to improve flexibility by increasing the range of motion of your joints. Although there is some debate as to whether or not stretching helps to decrease the risk of injury, it is generally assumed in the fitness industry that stretching is beneficial for everyone. Outlined below are some basic guidelines and techniques for improving your flexibility.

When should I stretch?

You may stretch every day if you wish, or you may stretch only on your workout days. Stretching can also be performed at any time of the day although the majority of people enjoy incorporating stretching before, during, or after a workout. Stretching during a workout helps to keep the muscle feeling "loose" and relaxed and may increase your joints' range of motion for the exercises that you are performing.

How should I stretch?

Before you do any stretching it is advisable to familiarize yourself with the exercises before beginning them. Do this by performing some light movements through the full range of motion of the joint you intend to stretch. Some prefer to do some light cardiovascular exercise for 5 – 10 minutes although this is not always necessary. It is important to remember to always let pain be your guide. Do not try and push a stretch to a range where it is painful for the muscles involved. You should feel the muscle under tension as you stretch it but it should not be uncomfortable. Proper flexibility training involves moving into the stretched position, holding that position for 10 to 15 seconds and then to try and move a little further into the stretch. After holding the new position for another 10 - 15 seconds, try to stretch a bit further. Continue this process until you can no longer move any furthur into the stretch. Depending on the muscle being stretched, you should be able to go a little bit further each time for a total of three times.

Putting together a stretching routine

Your stretching routine should incorporate at least one stretching exercise for each major muscle group. This would include stretches for the chest, upper back, lower back, shoulders, biceps, triceps, front thigh, rear thigh and calves. If you have tight muscles in certain areas that require special attention such as in the rotator cuff, hip flexors, hip rotators include a specific routine for that area as well. However, if you have the time it is a good idea to include as many muscle groups as possible. Unlike a weight training routine, it is not necessary to change stretching exercises every few months if you are progressing.

STRETCHES

CHEST STRETCH

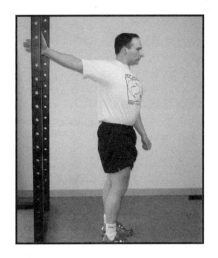

STARTING POSITION:
- With your arm straight, place the palm of your hand at neck level against a wall or a post that is to one side of you.
- Hold your head and chest high while keeping your back straight.

STRETCHING MOVEMENT:
- Slowly rotate your torso away from the wall or post by turning your shoulders, hips and feet towards the opposite side.

UPPER BACK STRETCH

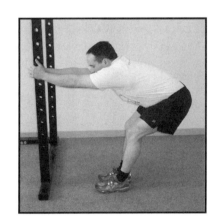

STARTING POSITION:
- Grasp a pole with both hands at approximately waist level that is securely attached to the floor or other heavy object that you can not move.
- Place both your feet close to the pole.
- Extend your hips backwards so that your body weight is shifted away from the pole.

STRETCHING MOVEMENT:
- Allow your upper back muscles to relax and your shoulders to pull forward as you lower your chest and head to the floor. You may bend your knees if you feel too much tension in the back of your thighs.

SINGLE ARM UPPER BACK STRETCH

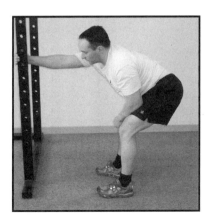

STARTING POSITION:
- Grasp a pole, one side of a doorframe, or other heavy object that you can not move with one hand.
- Place both your feet close to the pole.
- Extend your hips backwards so that your body weight is shifted away from the pole.

STRETCHING MOVEMENT:
- Allow your upper back muscles to relax and your shoulder to pull forward as you lower your chest and head to the floor. You may bend your knees if you feel too much tension in the backs of your thighs. At the lower portion of the movement twist your hips to the opposite side to extend the stretch furthur.

STRETCHING

LOWER BACK STRETCH

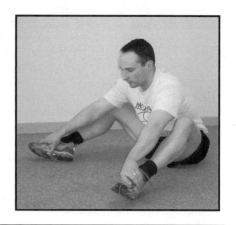

STARTING POSITION:
- Sit on the floor with your legs in front of you, your knees bent at a comfortable angle and your feet sideways on the floor positioned at least shoulder width apart.

STRETCHING MOVEMENT:
- Lean forward and grasp your feet while keeping your knees bent.
- Pull your torso down towards the floor using your arms.

SEATED LOWER BACK STRETCH

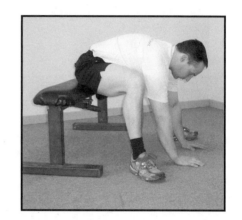

STARTING POSITION:
- Sit on the edge of a chair or exercise bench with your knees bent at a comfortable angle and your feet flat on the floor.

STRETCHING MOVEMENT:
- Lean forward allowing your torso to go between your legs and attempt to put the palms of your hands on the floor.
- For a greater stretch try placing your hands furthur out away from your body.

FRONT SHOULDER STRETCH

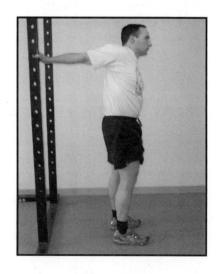

STARTING POSITION:
- With your arm straight, place the thumb side and inside knuckle of your hand at neck level against a wall or a post that is to one side of you.
- Hold your head and chest high while keeping your back straight.

STRETCHING MOVEMENT:
- Slowly rotate your torso away from the wall or post by turning your shoulders, hips and feet towards the opposite side.

STRETCHING

SIDE SHOULDER STRETCH

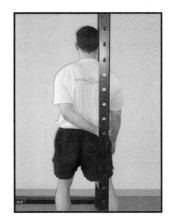

STARTING POSITION:
- Stand in front of a pole or door frame so that it is positioned directly behind you at the midline of your body.
- Reach behind and grasp the pole with a thumb up position at or just below belt level.

STRETCHING MOVEMENT:
- Allow your upper body to lean to the same side of the arm that is grasping the pole.

REAR SHOULDER STRETCH

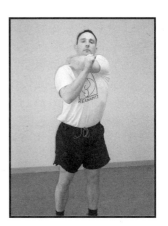

STARTING POSITION:
- Bend your arm at 90° and position your upper arm parallel to the floor. Push your shoulder forward allowing your upper back on that side to round.
- Cup your elbow with your other hand and support the weight of your arm.

STRETCHING MOVEMENT:
- Pull your arm across your upper chest and over your opposite shoulder.

ROTATOR CUFF STRETCH

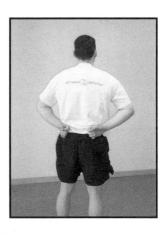

STARTING POSITION:
- Position both your hands behind your back. The backs of your hands should be placed on the outside of your waist but still behind your back.

STRETCHING MOVEMENT:
- Keeping your hands stationary, bring your elbows forward allowing your shoulders to rotate forward.
- Remember to hold you chest high.

OVERHEAD ROTATOR CUFF STRETCH

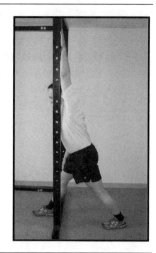

STARTING POSITION:
- With your arm straight, place the palm of your hand high above your head against a door frame or post that is positioned directly in front of your arm.
- Place the foot opposite your outstretched arm in front of your body.

STRETCHING MOVEMENT:
- Lean in towards the wall or pole, allowing your arm to stretch back. For a greater stretch, lean your body furthur down towards the floor.

LATERAL ROTATOR CUFF STRETCH

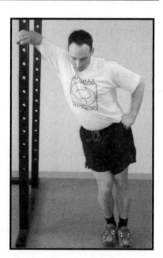

STARTING POSITION:
- Stand beside a wall place your forearm against a wall with your arm bent at 90°.
- Position your feet about 2 – 3 feet away from the wall. Your body should be at a slight angle to the floor with your shoulders and elbow positioned in a straight line.

STRETCHING MOVEMENT:
- Lean in towards the wall, allowing your arm to stretch upwards as your upper body moves down towards the floor. Bend your knees to help increase the range of motion.

INTERNAL ROTATOR CUFF STRETCH

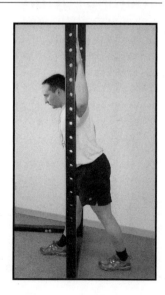

STARTING POSITION:
- With your arm bent at 90°, place your forearm vertically against a door frame or post with your elbow at the level of your shoulder.
- Place the foot opposite your shoulder that is being stretched in front of your body.

STRETCHING MOVEMENT:
- Lean your torso forward alongside the door frame or pole, allowing your upper arm to rotate back in relation to your body. For a greater stretch, lean your body furthur down towards the floor.

STRETCHING

BICEPS STRETCH

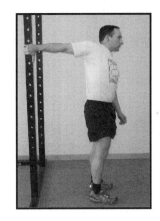

STARTING POSITION:
- With your arm straight, grasp a pole behind you so that your hand is positioned at chest or shoulder level with your thumb pointing down.
- Hold your head and chest high while keeping your back straight.

STRETCHING MOVEMENT:
- To stretch this muscle bring your hips forward so that your torso has a slight lean backwards.

TRICEPS STRETCH

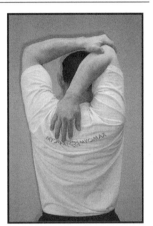

STARTING POSITION:
- Place one hand at the base of your neck so that your fingers are pointing down and your elbow pointing up.
- Place your other arm across the top of your head so that you can grasp your elbow. Keep your chin up.

STRETCHING MOVEMENT:
- To stretch this muscle pull your elbow towards the back of your head and opposite shoulder so that you feel the muscles stretch behind your upper arm.

FRONT THIGH STRETCH

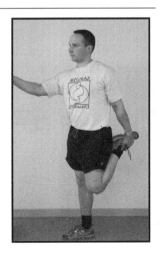

STARTING POSITION:
- While standing on one leg grasp the ankle of the opposite leg. To help with your balance you may wish to do this near a wall or other object.
- While keeping an upright position, place the knee of the bent leg beside the knee of the supporting leg. You can also do this stretch lying on one side on the floor.

STRETCHING MOVEMENT:
- While hanging onto your ankle, pull the leg slightly back and allow the hip of the same leg to thrust forward.

REAR THIGH STRETCH

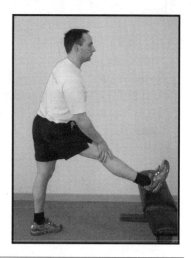

STARTING POSITION:
- Place the heel of one of your legs on a bench or a chair. Straighten your leg so that your knee is locked and the toe is pointing upwards.

STRETCHING MOVEMENT:
- While keeping your leg locked at the knee, lean forward holding your chest high so that your back is straight.

STANDING HIP FLEXOR STRETCH

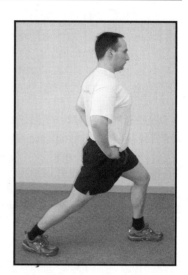

STARTING POSITION:
- Take a big step forward so that your front leg is several feet in front of the other.
- Position your body so that your hips and shoulders are aligned and facing forwards.
- Place both your hands on your hips.

STRETCHING MOVEMENT:
- While keeping your back leg straight, bend the knee of your forward leg as you lean your torso back slightly.
- You may wish to twist the hips slightly away from the back in order to achieve a better stretch. As long as your back leg stays locked at the knee, it does not matter if the heel of your back foot rises off the floor.

DEEP HIP FLEXOR STRETCH

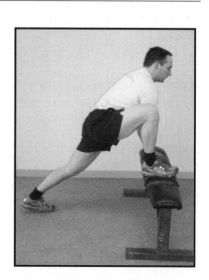

STARTING POSITION:
- Place one foot on top of an exercise bench or on the third step of a staircase.
- While keeping one foot on the bench, take a big step backwards so that your front leg is several feet in front of the back leg.
- Place both your hands for support on the portion of the bench on the inside of the foot.

STRETCHING MOVEMENT:
- While keeping your chest high bring the hips in towards the bench as you slightly roll the hip of the outstretched leg downwards. If you wish you can bend the knee of the outstretched leg in order to feel the stretch deep in the hip of the outstretched leg.

STRETCHING

BENCH HIP FLEXOR STRETCH

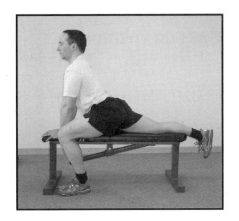

STARTING POSITION:

- Place one of your legs on top of a bench with your knee and foot pointing towards the floor. Place your other foot flat on the floor beside the bench and in front of your body so that when you bend the knee your hips are close to the bench.
- Make sure you keep the leg on top of the bench as straight as possible with the hip close to the bench.
- Place both your hands on the bench to support your upper body.

STRETCHING MOVEMENT:

- While keeping your hip on the bench, push your upper body away from the bench so your chest rises and your back arches upwards.
- To feel a greater stretch, roll the hip on the bench towards the floor.

SEATED OUTER HIP AND GLUTE STRETCH

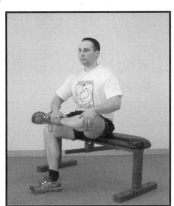

STARTING POSITION:

- Sit on the edge of a chair or bench so that your knees are bent at 90° with your feet flat on the floor. Cross one leg across your lap so that the ankle is directly above the knee and lower thigh.
- Place the hand on the side of the leg that is crossed on top of the side of the knee that is crossed.

STRETCHING MOVEMENT:

- While keeping your hand on the knee and applying pressure to hold the knee down and in position, lean forward keeping your chest up and your back straight so that you feel the stretch in the outside of the hip joint.

LYING OUTER HIP AND GLUTE STRETCH

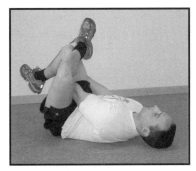

STARTING POSITION:

- Lie on the floor with one leg in the air bent at 90° so that the lower leg is parallel to the floor.
- Cross the opposite leg across your lap so that the ankle is resting just below the knee on the opposite leg.

STRETCHING MOVEMENT:

- Pull the thigh of the leg that is bent towards you with both hands positioned just below the ankle of the crossed leg.

STRETCHING

GLUTE AND HIP STRETCH

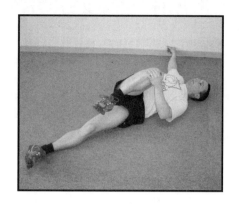

STARTING POSITION:
- Lie on the floor with one leg straight and the other leg bent at 90° with your lower leg parallel to the floor.
- Place your opposite hand just below the knee of the bent leg.

STRETCHING MOVEMENT:
- Pull the knee of the bent leg in towards and across your upper body so that you feel the stretch in the lower portion of the back of the hips.

CALF STRETCH

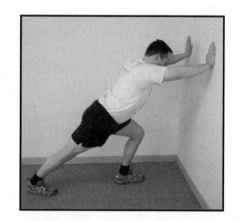

STARTING POSITION:
- Stand facing a wall and take a big step backwards and place the heel of the foot flat on the floor. Bend the front leg and support yourself with your hands against the wall.

STRETCHING MOVEMENT:
- Bend the front leg so that the knee moves forward so that you feel the stretch in the back of the lower leg.
- Make sure the heel of the back leg always touches the floor.

WALL CALF STRETCH

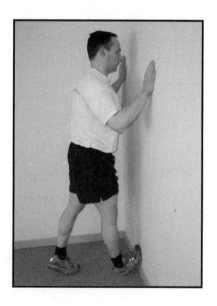

STARTING POSITION:
- Stand facing a wall, pole, or step. Place the ball and toes of one of your feet against the wall several inches above the floor so that the heel can still touch the ground.

STRETCHING MOVEMENT:
- Move your upper body in close to the wall or pole, making sure that the heel of the leg that is being stretched does not slip away from the wall.
- Make sure the heel of the foot touching the wall always touches the floor.

LYING OBLIQUE AND LOWER BACK STRETCH

STARTING POSITION:
- Lie on the floor with one leg straight and the other leg bent at 90° with your lower leg parallel to the floor.
- Place your opposite hand to the leg that is bent on the outside of the knee. Extend your arm out to the side to help you balance.

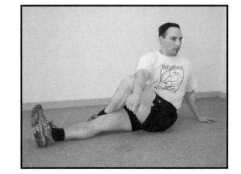

STRETCHING MOVEMENT:
- Pull the knee of the bent leg towards the floor on the side of the straight leg. Make sure you keep your leg bent at 90°.
- As you rotate your hips and leg to one side, try and keep both shoulders on the ground at all times.

SITTING OBLIQUE AND LOWER BACK STRETCH

STARTING POSITION:
- Sit on the floor with one leg straight while the other leg crosses over the thigh of the straight leg. The foot of the leg that is bent should be positioned beside the knee of the straight leg.
- Twist your torso so that the opposite arm of the bent leg is braced against the thigh of the bent leg. Your other arm should be extended behind you to help you twist and keep your balance.

STRETCHING MOVEMENT:
- Try and twist your torso and your shoulders as far as you can to the side of the bent leg.
- To help get a better stretch, push off of the bent leg.
- Try and keep both your hips on the floor at all times.

REAR VIEW

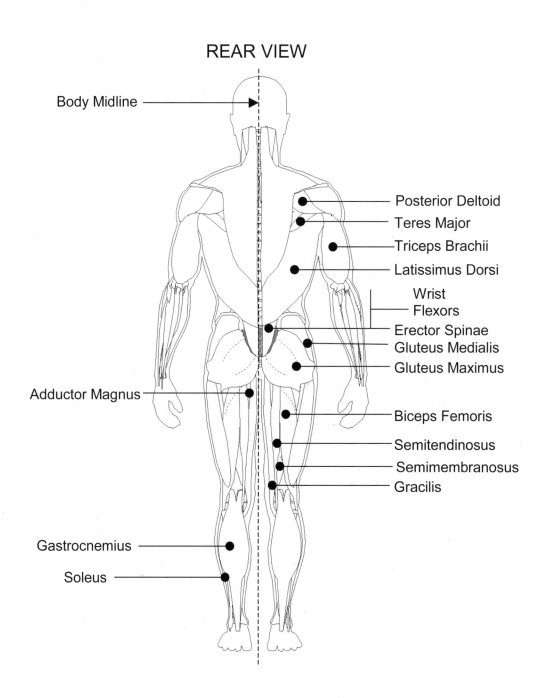

Body Midline

Posterior Deltoid
Teres Major
Triceps Brachii
Latissimus Dorsi
Wrist
Flexors
Erector Spinae
Gluteus Medialis
Gluteus Maximus

Adductor Magnus

Biceps Femoris

Semitendinosus
Semimembranosus
Gracilis

Gastrocnemius

Soleus

FRONT VIEW

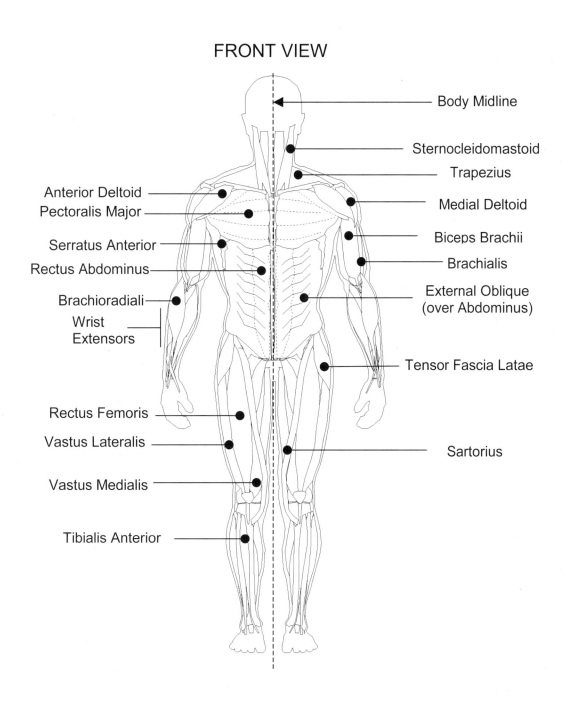

Body Midline

Sternocleidomastoid

Trapezius

Anterior Deltoid

Medial Deltoid

Pectoralis Major

Biceps Brachii

Serratus Anterior

Brachialis

Rectus Abdominus

External Oblique
(over Abdominus)

Brachioradiali

Wrist
Extensors

Tensor Fascia Latae

Rectus Femoris

Vastus Lateralis

Sartorius

Vastus Medialis

Tibialis Anterior

MUSCLE ANATOMY

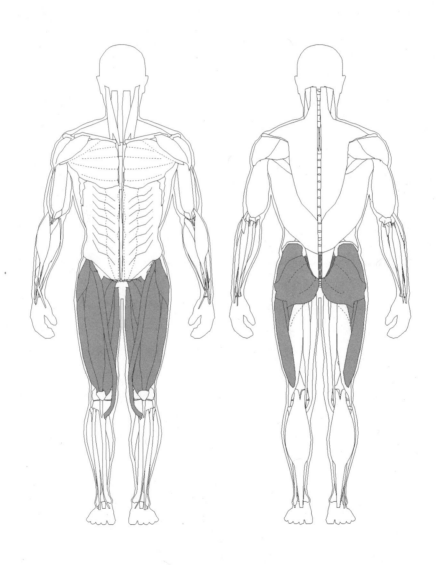

SQUATS

MAJOR MUSCLES IN USE:

Vastus Lateralis, Rectus Femoris, Vastus Medialis, Gluteus Maximus, Biceps Femoris, Semitendinosus, Semimembranosus, Erector Spinae

STARTING POSITION:

- Standing in front of a squat rack, place the bar across the top of the back of your shoulders so that the bar rests on the lower part of your trapezius muscle.
- Step back from the rack and position your feet shoulder width apart with your toes pointing slightly outwards.
- Look straight ahead with your abdominal and lower back muscles tensed.
- You should be standing with your chest up, back slightly arched, and leaning slightly forward from the waist.

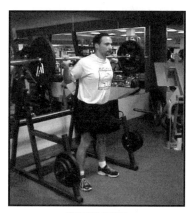

START

EXERCISE MOVEMENT:

- Keeping your chest up and looking straight ahead, lower yourself into a squatting position by pushing your hips out and bending at the knees.
- Your knees should follow their natural path out over the tops of your feet.
- Keeping your chest up, lean forward slightly at the waist as your thighs approach a position parallel to the floor.
- Once your thighs are parallel to the floor, reverse the motion so that you finish in the standing position.

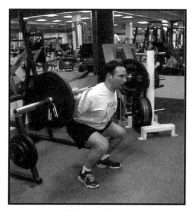

FINISH

EXERCISE TECHNIQUE POINTS:

- Do not round your back at any time during the exercise.
- Do not lean forward excessively during the descent phase so that you feel the muscles tightening more in the lower back than in the thighs.
- Think of sitting down in a chair as you begin the descent phase, by leading the motion with your hips instead of the knees.
- Do not allow your heels to come off the floor. To stop your heels from coming off the floor, lead a bit more with the hips.
- Do not allow your hips to become lower than your knees.
- If you find it difficult to balance, you may place a thin board or weight plate under your heels.

DIFFICULTY -	H	H	H
♂ STARTING WEIGHT - 85			
♀ STARTING WEIGHT - 55			

DUMBBELL SQUATS

MAJOR MUSCLES IN USE:
Vastus Lateralis, Rectus Femoris, Vastus Medialis, Gluteus Maximus, Biceps Femoris, Semitendinosus, Semimembranosus, Erector Spinae

STARTING POSITION:
- Grasp a pair of moderately heavy dumbbells and hold them at your sides.
- Position your feet about shoulder width apart with your toes pointing slightly outwards.
- Look straight ahead with your abdominal and lower back muscles tensed.
- You should be standing straight with your chest up and your back slightly arched.

EXERCISE MOVEMENT:
- Keeping your chest up and looking straight ahead, lower yourself into a squatting position by pushing your hips out and bending at the knees.
- Your knees should follow their natural path out over the tops of your feet.
- Keeping your chest up, lean forward slightly at the waist as your thighs approach a position parallel to the floor.
- Once your thighs are parallel to the floor, reverse the motion so that you finish in the standing position.

EXERCISE TECHNIQUE POINTS:
- Do not round your back at any time during the exercise.
- You may have to lean a bit farther forward than you normally would in doing squats in order to do the motion properly.
- As you begin the descent phase, think of sitting down in a chair by leading the motion with your hips instead of the knees.
- Do not allow your heels to come off the floor. If your heels do come off the floor, make sure to lead a bit more with the hips. You could also elevate your heels slightly by placing them on a thin board or weight plates.

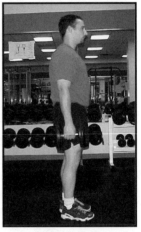

START

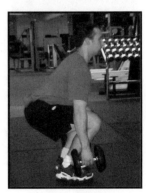

FINISH

DIFFICULTY -	⊢⊣	⊢⊣	⊢⊣
♂ STARTING WEIGHT - 20			
♀ STARTING WEIGHT - 10			

WIDE STANCE SQUATS

MAJOR MUSCLES IN USE:

Vastus Lateralis, Rectus Femoris, Vastus Medialis, Gluteus Maximus, Biceps Femoris, Semitendinosus, Semimembranosus, Erector Spinae, Gluteus Medius, Adductor Magnus, Gracilis

STARTING POSITION:
- Standing in front of a squat rack, place the bar across the lower portion of the back of your shoulders.
- Step back from the rack and position your feet about a foot wider than shoulder width apart with your toes pointing outwards.
- Look straight ahead with your abdominal and lower back muscles tensed.
- You should be standing with your chest up, back slightly arched, and leaning slightly forward at the waist.

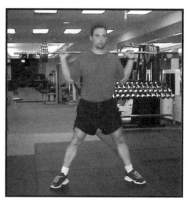

START

EXERCISE MOVEMENT:
- Keeping your chest up and looking straight ahead, bend at the knees and begin to lower yourself into a squatting position.
- Your knees should follow their natural path out over the top of your feet .
- Lean forward very slightly at the waist, keeping your chest out, as you squat down and your thighs approach a position parallel to the floor.
- Once the angle between your calves and your thighs reaches 90°, reverse the motion so that you finish back in the standing position.

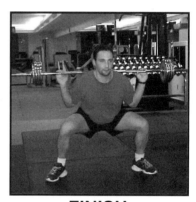

FINISH

EXERCISE TECHNIQUE POINTS:
- Do not round your back at any time during the exercise.
- As you begin the descent phase, think of sitting down in a chair by leading the motion with your hips instead of the knees.
- Be careful not to go too low as this can put extra strain on your hip muscles.
- Do not allow your heels to come off the floor. If your heels do come off the floor, think of sitting back even farther and push down with your heels.

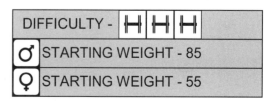

DIFFICULTY -	H H H
♂ STARTING WEIGHT - 85	
♀ STARTING WEIGHT - 55	

SUMO SQUATS

MAJOR MUSCLES IN USE:

Vastus Lateralis, Rectus Femoris, Vastus Medialis, Gluteus Maximus, Biceps Femoris, Semitendinosus, Semimembranosus, Gluteus Medius, Adductor Magnus, Gracilis

STARTING POSITION:

- Straddle either a barbell or a heavy dumbbell by placing your feet at least 3 - 4 feet apart with your toes pointing outwards. You may wish to stand on two low benches in order to increase the range of motion.
- Bend your legs so that you can grasp the barbell. Your hands should be placed about 2 feet apart or you can grasp the end of the dumbbell with both hands.

EXERCISE MOVEMENT:

- Keeping your chest up and looking straight ahead, slowly stand up until your legs are straight.
- Once you reach a standing position, reverse the movement so that you lower the weight back down towards the ground.

EXERCISE TECHNIQUE POINTS:

- Do not round your back at any time during the exercise.
- As you begin the descent phase, think of sitting down in a chair by leading the motion with your hips instead of the knees.
- Do not allow your knees to rotate inwards or bend in as you lift or lower the weight.

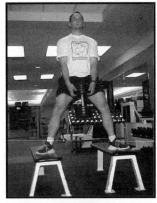

START

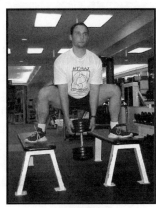

FINISH

DIFFICULTY -	H H H	
♂	STARTING WEIGHT - 35	
♀	STARTING WEIGHT - 20	

BODYBUILDER SQUATS

MAJOR MUSCLES IN USE:

Vastus Lateralis, Rectus Femoris, Vastus Medialis, Gluteus Maximus, Biceps Femoris, Semitendinosus, Semimembranosus, Erector Spinae

STARTING POSITION:

- Standing in front of a squat rack, place the bar across the back of your shoulders so that the bar is resting on the high portion of your trapezius muscles. The bar should still be below your most prominent neck bone (C7).
- Step back from the rack and position your feet about 8 inches apart with your toes pointing straight ahead.
- Look straight ahead with your abdominal and lower back muscles tensed.
- You should be standing with your chest up, back slightly arched, leaning slightly forward.

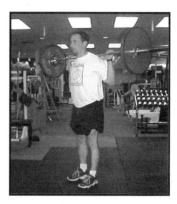

START

EXERCISE MOVEMENT:

- Keeping your chest up and looking straight ahead, bend at the hips and knees and begin to lower yourself into a squatting position.
- You should be leading with the hips as if you were about to sit down on a chair.
- As your thighs approach a position parallel to the floor, lean forward at the waist.
- Once your thighs are parallel to the floor or your knee angle is less than 90°, reverse the motion so that you finish back in the standing position.

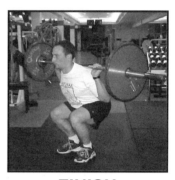

FINISH

EXERCISE TECHNIQUE POINTS:

- Do not round your back at any time during the exercise.
- Do not lean forward excessively during the descent phase. You should not feel the muscles tightening more in the lower back than in the thighs.
- Do not allow your heels to come off the floor. If your heels do come off the floor, make sure to lead a little more with the hips.
- Do not allow your hips to become lower than your knees.

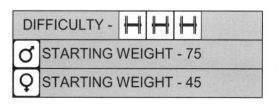

DIFFICULTY -	⊢ ⊢ ⊢	
♂	STARTING WEIGHT - 75	
♀	STARTING WEIGHT - 45	

FRONT THIGH AND HIP EXERCISES   43

BARBELL HACK SQUATS

MAJOR MUSCLES IN USE:
Vastus Lateralis, Rectus Femoris, Vastus Medialis, Gluteus Maximus, Biceps Femoris, Semitendinosus, Semimembranosus

STARTING POSITION:
- While standing in front of a barbell, position your feet about shoulder-width apart with your toes pointing forward.
- Squat down and grasp the barbell with an overhand grip. Your hands should be about shoulder-width apart.
- Look straight ahead with your abdominal and lower back muscles tensed.

EXERCISE MOVEMENT:
- Lift the barbell by standing up while keeping your arms straight and your chest up. When you are standing the barbell should be resting against the backs of your thighs, just below the buttocks.
- Lean forward slightly at the waist, keeping your chest out, as you squat back down to the starting position.
- Your knees should follow a natural path out over the tops of your feet.
- Once the barbell touches the floor, repeat the motion for the desired number of repetitions.

EXERCISE TECHNIQUE POINTS:
- Do not round your back at any time during the exercise.
- Do not lean forward excessively during the descent phase so that you feel the muscles tightening more in the lower back than in the thighs.
- As you begin the descent phase, think of sitting down in a chair by leading the motion with your hips instead of the knees.
- You may wish to elevate the heels by placing a board or a plate under each foot to help you keep your balance and your heels in contact with the floor.

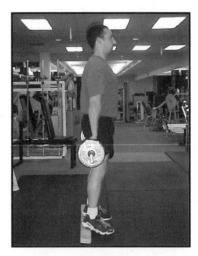

START

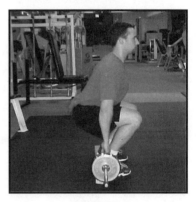

FINISH

DIFFICULTY -	H H H H	
♂	STARTING WEIGHT - 55	
♀	STARTING WEIGHT - 25	

FRONT THIGH AND HIP EXERCISES

FRONT SQUATS

MAJOR MUSCLES IN USE:

Vastus Lateralis, Rectus Femoris, Vastus Medialis, Gluteus Maximus, Biceps Femoris, Semitendinosus, Semimembranosus, Erector Spinae

STARTING POSITION:

- Standing in front of a squat rack, place the bar across the top of your chest right at the base of your neck.
- Cross your arms over the bar so that each hand is over the top of the opposite shoulder. Your upper arms should be parallel to the floor with your elbows held high at all times.
- Step back from the rack and position your feet shoulder-width apart with your toes pointing slightly outwards.
- Look up with your abdominal and lower back muscles tensed while keeping your chest high.

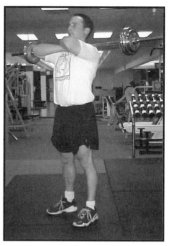

START

EXERCISE MOVEMENT:

- Keeping your chest high and looking up, begin the motion by leading with the hips and bending at the knees to lower yourself into a squatting position.
- Your knees should follow their natural path out over the top of your feet.
- Try and stay as upright as possible as you squat down.
- Once your thighs are parallel to the floor reverse the motion so that you finish back in the starting position.

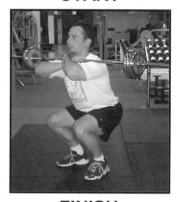

FINISH

EXERCISE TECHNIQUE POINTS:

- Do not round your back at any time during the exercise.
- Do not lean forward excessively during the descent phase. You should not feel the muscles tense more in the lower back than in the thighs.
- As you begin the descent phase, think of sitting down in a chair by leading the motion with your hips instead of the knees.
- By holding your elbows high, you will keep the weight secure.

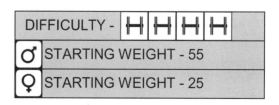

DIFFICULTY -	H H H H
♂ STARTING WEIGHT - 55	
♀ STARTING WEIGHT - 25	

ONE LEGGED SQUAT

MAJOR MUSCLES IN USE:

Vastus Lateralis, Rectus Femoris, Vastus Medialis, Gluteus Maximus, Biceps Femoris, Semitendinosus, Semimembranosus, Erector Spinae

STARTING POSITION:

- Grasp a pair of moderately heavy dumbbells and hold them at your sides.
- Position your front leg about one foot in front of your body.
- Place your other foot about two feet behind you so that it is resting on a bench with your knee bent and the sole of the foot facing upwards.
- Tense your abdominal and lower back muscles.

EXERCISE MOVEMENT:

- Keeping your chest high and looking straight ahead, begin the motion by lowering yourself by bending the front knee.
- As you lower yourself, lean forward to shift your body weight to the front leg. Your back leg should not contribute to the lifting or lowering of the weight.
- Your front knee should follow its natural path out over the top of your foot which should be pointed straight ahead. Your leading knee should not cross over the tips of your toes.
- Once your thigh is parallel to the floor, reverse the motion so that you finish back in the starting position.

EXERCISE TECHNIQUE POINTS:

- Do not round your back at any time during the exercise.
- Use your back leg to help balance but not to help lift the weight.
- If you have trouble keeping your balance, try taking a wider than shoulder-width stance, or a longer stride.

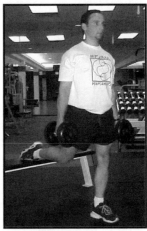

START

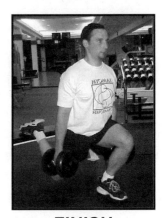

FINISH

DIFFICULTY -	H	H	H	H
♂	STARTING WEIGHT – no weight			
♀	STARTING WEIGHT – no weight			

FRONT THIGH AND HIP EXERCISES 46

STEP-UPS

MAJOR MUSCLES IN USE:
Vastus Lateralis, Rectus Femoris, Vastus Medialis, Gluteus Maximus, Biceps Femoris, Semitendinosus, Semimembranosus, Erector Spinae

STARTING POSITION:
- Grasp a pair of moderately heavy dumbbells and hold them at your sides.
- Stand perpendicular to a low bench or step and place one of your feet on the bench so that your thigh is parallel to the floor.
- Tense your abdominal and lower back muscles.

EXERCISE MOVEMENT:
- Keeping your chest high and looking straight ahead, begin the motion by stepping up on the bench with your other foot so that your forward thigh is doing most of the lifting.
- As you step onto the bench, lean forward to shift your body weight to the front leg. Your back leg should not contribute to the lifting of the weight.
- Your front knee should follow its natural path out over the top of your foot which should be pointed straight ahead. Your leading knee should not cross over the tips of your toes.
- Once you are standing on the bench or step with both feet beside each other, reverse the motion back to the starting so that you step back leaving the same foot on the bench that you began with.

EXERCISE TECHNIQUE POINTS:
- Do not round your back at any time during the exercise.
- Use your back leg to help balance but not to help lift the weight.
- If you have trouble keeping your balance, try taking a wider than shoulder-width stance or try a lower step or bench.
- Lower yourself slowly back to the starting position to avoid excessive stress on the knees and ankles.

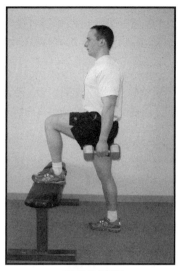

START

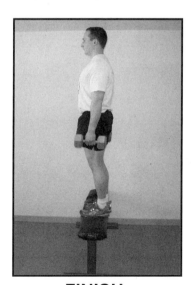

FINISH

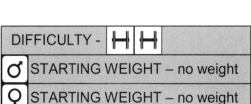

DIFFICULTY -	H H	
♂	STARTING WEIGHT – no weight	
♀	STARTING WEIGHT – no weight	

LATERAL STEP-UPS

MAJOR MUSCLES IN USE:

Vastus Lateralis, Rectus Femoris, Vastus Medialis, Gluteus Maximus, Biceps Femoris, Semitendinosus, Semimembranosus, Adductor Magnus

STARTING POSITION:
- Grasp a pair of moderately heavy dumbbells and hold them at your sides.
- Stand beside a low bench or step and place one foot in the middle of the bench so that your thigh is parallel to the floor.
- Tense your abdominal and lower back muscles.

EXERCISE MOVEMENT:
- Keeping your chest high and looking straight ahead, begin the motion by stepping up on the bench with your other foot so that your forward thigh is doing most of the lifting.
- As you step onto the bench, lean forward to shift your body weight to the front leg. Your back leg should not contribute to the lifting of the weight.
- Your front knee should follow its natural path out over the top of your foot which should be pointed straight ahead. Your leading knee should not cross over the tips of your toes.
- Once you are standing on the bench or step with both feet beside each other, reverse the motion back to the starting so that you step back leaving the same foot on the bench that you began with.

EXERCISE TECHNIQUE POINTS:
- Do not round your back at any time during the exercise.
- Use your back leg to help balance but not to help lift the weight.
- If you have trouble keeping your balance, try taking a wider than shoulder-width stance or try a lower step or bench.
- Lower yourself slowly back to the starting position to avoid excessive stress on the knees and ankles.

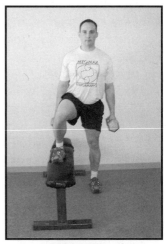

START

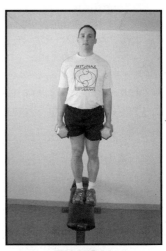

FINISH

DIFFICULTY -	H	H	
♂	STARTING WEIGHT - no weight		
♀	STARTING WEIGHT - no weight		

SPLIT SQUATS

MAJOR MUSCLES IN USE:

Vastus Lateralis, Rectus Femoris, Vastus Medialis, Gluteus Maximus, Biceps Femoris, Semitendinosus, Semimembranosus, Erector Spinae

STARTING POSITION:

- Grasp a pair of moderately heavy dumbbells and hold them at your sides.
- While facing forward, place one foot a distance of about 3 – 4 feet in front of the other foot.
- Your feet should be about shoulder width apart. Tense your abdominal and lower back muscles.

EXERCISE MOVEMENT:

- Keeping your chest held high and looking straight ahead, lower yourself by bending the front knee.
- As you lower yourself, your back knee should bend slightly and your heel should rise up off the floor as you move farther down into the movement.
- Your front knee should follow its natural path out over the top of your foot (which should be pointed straight ahead). However, your knee should not extend beyond the tips of the toes.
- Once your thigh reaches a position parallel to the floor or your knee comes very close to the floor, reverse the motion so that you finish back in the standing position.

EXERCISE TECHNIQUE POINTS:

- Do not round your back at any time during the exercise.
- Do not lean forward excessively during the descent phase. You should not feel the muscles tighten more in the lower back than in the thighs.

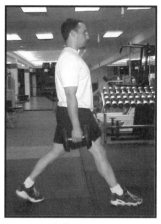

START

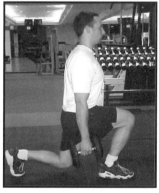

FINISH

DIFFICULTY -	⊢∣ ⊢∣ ⊢∣	
♂	STARTING WEIGHT - 15	
♀	STARTING WEIGHT - 10	

FRONT THIGH AND HIP EXERCISES 49

FORWARD LUNGES

MAJOR MUSCLES IN USE:

Vastus Lateralis, Rectus Femoris, Vastus Medialis, Gluteus Maximus, Biceps Femoris, Semitendinosus, Semimembranosus, Erector Spinae

STARTING POSITION:

- Grasp a pair of moderately heavy dumbbells and hold them at your sides.
- Position yourself facing forward with your feet about shoulder width apart and your toes pointing forward.
- Tense your abdominal and lower back muscles.

EXERCISE MOVEMENT:

- Keeping your chest high and looking straight ahead, begin the motion by taking a large step (about 3 - 4 feet in length) forward.
- As you lunge forward, your back knee should bend slightly. Your heel should rise up off the floor as you move into the step.
- Your leading knee should follow its natural path out over the top of your foot (which should be pointed straight ahead). However, this knee should not go any farther than the tips of your toes.
- Once your thigh reaches a position parallel to the floor, or your knee comes very close to the floor, reverse the motion so that you finish back in the starting position.

EXERCISE TECHNIQUE POINTS:

- Do not round your back at any time during the exercise.
- Do not lean forward excessively during the descent phase. You should not feel the muscles tighten more in the lower back than in the thighs.
- If you have trouble keeping your balance, try taking a wider stance, or try to lunge a little farther by taking a larger step.

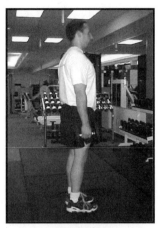

START

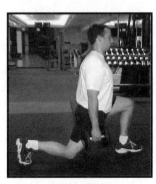

FINISH

DIFFICULTY -	⊢	⊢	⊢	⊢
♂	STARTING WEIGHT - 15			
♀	STARTING WEIGHT - 10			

WALKING LUNGES

MAJOR MUSCLES IN USE:

Vastus Lateralis, Rectus Femoris, Vastus Medialis, Gluteus Maximus, Biceps Femoris, Semitendinosus, Semimembranosus, Erector Spinae

STARTING POSITION:
- Grasp a pair of dumbbells and hold them at your sides.
- Face towards an area long enough to allow room for the exercise.
- Your feet should be close together with toes pointed forward.
- Tense your abdominal and lower back muscles.

EXERCISE MOVEMENT:
- Keeping your chest high and looking straight ahead, begin the motion by taking a large step (about 3 - 4 feet in length) forward.
- As you "lunge" forward, your back knee should slightly bend; your heel should come up off the floor as you move into the step.
- Your front knee should follow its natural path out over the top of your foot which should be pointed straight ahead. However, your lead knee should not extend any farther than the tips of your toes.
- Once your thigh is parallel to the floor or your back knee is about 1 inch above the floor, lean forward slightly and finish the forward stride as if rising out of a very large step.
- Once you are standing again, take another large stride as before with the opposite leg. Continue lunging until all the necessary repetitions are done for each leg.

EXERCISE TECHNIQUE POINTS:
- Do not round your back at any time during the exercise.
- If you have trouble keeping your balance try taking a wider stance or try to lunge a little farther.

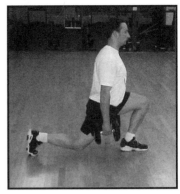

START

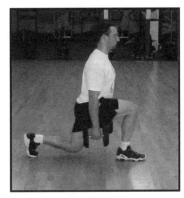

FINISH

DIFFICULTY -	H	H	H
♂ STARTING WEIGHT - no weight			
♀ STARTING WEIGHT - no weight			

FRONT THIGH AND HIP EXERCISES

REVERSE LUNGES

MAJOR MUSCLES IN USE:

Vastus Lateralis, Rectus Femoris, Vastus Medialis, Gluteus Maximus, Biceps Femoris, Semitendinosus, Semimembranosus, Erector Spinae

STARTING POSITION:
- Grasp a pair of dumbbells and hold them at your sides.
- Position yourself facing forward with your feet about shoulder-width apart, toes pointing forward.
- Tense your abdominal and lower back muscles.

EXERCISE MOVEMENT:
- Keeping your chest high and looking straight ahead, begin the motion by taking a large step (about 3 - 4 feet in length) backwards with either your left or your right foot.
- As you lunge backwards, your front knee will bend and your back foot should land on the ball of the foot with your heel off the ground.
- Both legs should bend at the knees at the same time as you lower yourself into the lunge position.
- Once your thigh reaches a position that is parallel to the floor, or your knee comes very close to the floor, reverse the motion so that you finish back in the starting position.

EXERCISE TECHNIQUE POINTS:
- Do not round your back at any time during the exercise.
- Do not lean forward excessively during the descent phase. You should feel the muscles tense more in the thighs than the lower back.
- If you have trouble keeping your balance try taking a wider than shoulder-width stance, or try to lunge a little farther.

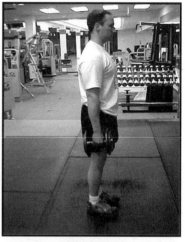

START

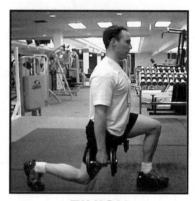

FINISH

DIFFICULTY - H H H H		
♂	STARTING WEIGHT - 15	
♀	STARTING WEIGHT - 10	

FRONT THIGH AND HIP EXERCISES 52

SIDE LUNGES

MAJOR MUSCLES IN USE:
Vastus Lateralis, Rectus Femoris, Vastus Medialis, Gluteus Maximus, Gluteus Medius, Adductor Magnus, Gracilis

STARTING POSITION:
- Standing in front of a squat rack, place the bar across the back of your shoulders with the bar resting on the lower portion of your trapezius muscles.
- Step several paces back from the squat rack, so that you are clear of the rack. Position yourself facing forward with your feet about shoulder-width apart, toes pointing slightly outwards.
- Tense your abdominal and lower back muscles.

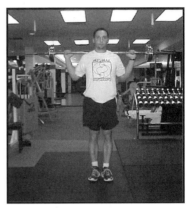

START

EXERCISE MOVEMENT:
- Keeping your chest high and looking straight ahead, begin the motion by taking a large step (about 3 - 4 feet in length) to the side with either your left or your right leg.
- As you step to the side, your stationary leg should remain straight with your foot on the ground and pointing slightly outwards. Your stepping leg should land with its foot pointing outwards so that you can bend at the knee until the thigh is parallel to the floor. The knee should follow its natural path out over the top of your foot. The knee of the lunging leg should not cross over the end of your toes.
- Try and stay as upright as possible as you lunge to the side.
- Once your thigh reaches a parallel position to the floor, powerfully reverse the motion so that you finish back in the starting position.

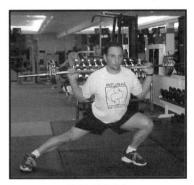

FINISH

EXERCISE TECHNIQUE POINTS:
- Do not round your back at any time during the exercise.
- Think of sitting back as you approach the bottom portion of the lunge.

DIFFICULTY -	H	H	H	H
♂ STARTING WEIGHT - 25				
♀ STARTING WEIGHT - no weight				

FRONT THIGH AND HIP EXERCISES   53

CABLE LEG ADDUCTION

MAJOR MUSCLES IN USE:
Gracilis, Adductor Magnus

STARTING POSITION:
- Stand sideways about 3 feet in front of a machine equipped with a low pulley apparatus. The ankle of your leg nearest to the pulley machine should be firmly attached to the cable with a strap.
- The leg to be exercised should be extended to the side so that you can feel a slight stretch in the inner thigh muscles. It may help to stand on a low platform so that your foot does not drag on the floor.
- Your weight should be centered over the non-exercising leg. It may be advisable to hang onto a chair or other structure to help keep your balance.

EXERCISE MOVEMENT:
- Keeping both legs straight, begin by pulling your attached ankle towards and slightly in front of the supporting leg. Continue pulling until your thighs touch and slightly cross over each other.
- Reverse the motion slowly back to the starting position and repeat for the scheduled number of repetitions. When finished perform the same exercise on the other leg.

EXERCISE TECHNIQUE POINTS:
- Stand tall and remember to keep your exercising leg straight.
- Try not to lean to one side in order to finish your repetitions.

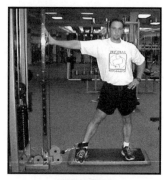

START

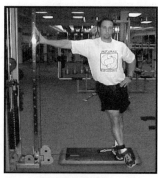

FINISH

DIFFICULTY -	⊢ ⊢ ⊢
♂ STARTING WEIGHT - 20	
♀ STARTING WEIGHT - 10	

CABLE LEG ABDUCTION

MAJOR MUSCLES IN USE:
Gluteus Medialis

STARTING POSITION:
- Stand sideways about 2 feet in front of a machine equipped with a low pulley apparatus. The ankle of your farthest leg should be firmly attached to the cable with a strap.
- The exercising leg should be slightly crossed in front of the supporting leg so that you can feel a slight stretch in the side of the hip furthest from the machine. You should also be standing on a slight platform in order that your foot does not drag on the floor.
- Your weight should be centered over the non-exercising leg and it may be advisable to hang onto a chair or other structure to help keep your balance.

EXERCISE MOVEMENT:
- Keeping the leg straight, begin by moving your attached ankle away from the machine. Continue bringing the leg out to the side until your leg is as far out as possible without leaning your torso towards the machine.
- Reverse the motion slowly back to the starting position and continue for the scheduled number of repetitions. When finished, perform the same exercise on the supporting leg.

EXERCISE TECHNIQUE POINTS:
- Stand tall and remember to keep your exercising leg straight.
- Try not to lean to one side in order to finish your repetitions.

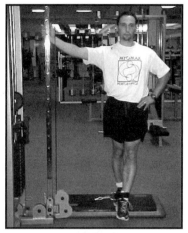

START

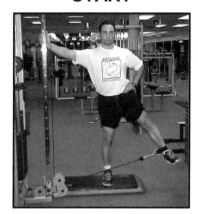

FINISH

DIFFICULTY -	⊢ ⊢ ⊩		
♂	STARTING WEIGHT - 20		
♀	STARTING WEIGHT - 10		

HIP FLEXION

MAJOR MUSCLES IN USE:
Tensor Fascia Latae, Rectus Femoris

STARTING POSITION:
- Stand with your back facing the front of a machine equipped with a low pulley apparatus. The ankle of the exercising leg should be firmly attached to the cable with a strap.
- The exercising leg should be slightly extended behind the supporting leg so that you can feel a slight stretch in the front of the hip. You should also be standing on a slight platform in order that your foot does not drag on the floor.
- You should be leaning slightly forward with your weight centered over the non-exercising leg. It may be advisable to hang onto a chair or other structure to help in keeping your balance.

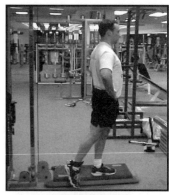

START

EXERCISE MOVEMENT:
- Begin by bending at the knee of the attached leg and lifting it forward and as high as possible as if you were climbing a staircase.
- Continue bringing the leg up as high as you can or until you begin to feel that your supporting leg is starting to bend.
- Reverse the motion slowly back to the starting position and repeat for the scheduled number of repetitions. When finished, perform the same exercise on the supporting leg.

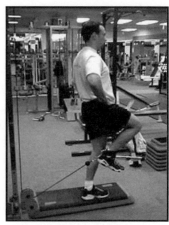

FINISH

EXERCISE TECHNIQUE POINTS:
- Lean forward slightly while maintaining a straight back.
- Do not allow the supporting leg to bend at the knee as you are reaching the top of the exercise motion.

DIFFICULTY -	⊢	⊢
♂	STARTING WEIGHT - 25	
♀	STARTING WEIGHT - 15	

FRONT THIGH AND HIP EXERCISES

STRAIGHT LEG HIP FLEXION

MAJOR MUSCLES IN USE:
  Tensor Fascia Latae, Rectus Femoris

STARTING POSITION:
- Position yourself with your back facing the front of a machine equipped with a low pulley apparatus. The ankle of the exercising leg should be firmly attached to the cable.
- The exercising leg should be placed slightly behind the supporting leg so that you can feel a slight stretch in the front of the hip. You should also be standing on a low platform so that your foot does not drag on the floor.
- You should lean forward slightly with your weight centered over the non-exercising leg. It may be advisable to hang onto a chair or other structure to help you keep your balance.

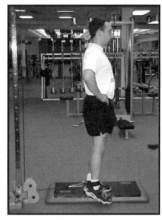
START

EXERCISE MOVEMENT:
- Keeping the exercising leg straight and locked at the knee, begin by moving the attached ankle forward as if you were kicking a ball. Continue bringing the leg forward until you feel your supporting leg begin to bend at the knee.
- Reverse the motion slowly back to the starting position and repeat for the scheduled number of repetitions. When finished, reverse legs and perform the same movement.

EXERCISE TECHNIQUE POINTS:
- Lean forward slightly while maintaining a straight back.
- Do not allow the supporting leg to bend at the knee as you near the top of the exercise motion.

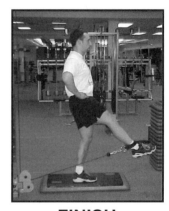
FINISH

DIFFICULTY - ⊢⊣ ⊢⊣	
♂	STARTING WEIGHT - 20
♀	STARTING WEIGHT - 10

FRONT THIGH AND HIP EXERCISES 57

LYING STRAIGHT LEG CABLE HIP FLEXION

MAJOR MUSCLES IN USE:
Tensor Fascia Latae, Rectus Femoris

STARTING POSITION:
- Position yourself on your back with your feet facing the front of a machine equipped with a low pulley apparatus. The ankle of the exercising leg should be firmly attached to the cable.
- The exercising leg should be placed directly beside the opposite leg with the heel touching the ground.
- Place your hands beside your body to help stabilize and to prevent yourself from moving forward. It may be advisable to hang onto a heavy weight chair or other structure to help you keep your balance and to remain stationary.

EXERCISE MOVEMENT:
- Keeping the exercising leg straight and locked at the knee, begin by moving the attached ankle upwards away from the floor as if you were kicking a ball over your head. Continue bringing the leg forward until you feel your supporting leg begin to bend at the knee.
- Reverse the motion slowly back to the starting position and repeat for the scheduled number of repetitions. When finished, reverse legs and perform the same movement.

EXERCISE TECHNIQUE POINTS:
- Keep your abdominal muscles tensed to help prevent your pelvis from moving.
- Do not allow the supporting leg to bend at the knee as you near the top of the exercise motion.

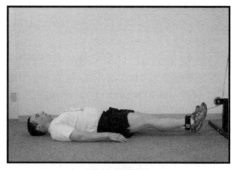

START

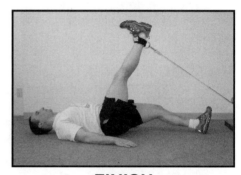

FINISH

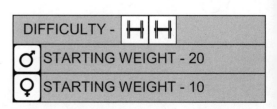

DIFFICULTY - ⊢⊢	
♂	STARTING WEIGHT - 20
♀	STARTING WEIGHT - 10

LYING CABLE HIP FLEXION

MAJOR MUSCLES IN USE:
Tensor Fascia Latae, Rectus Femoris

STARTING POSITION:
- Position yourself on your back with your feet facing the front of a machine equipped with a low pulley apparatus. The ankle of the exercising leg should be firmly attached to the cable.
- The exercising leg should be placed directly beside the opposite leg with the heel touching the ground.
- Place your hands beside your body to help stabilize and to prevent yourself from moving forward. It may be advisable to hang onto a heavy weight chair or other structure to help you keep your balance and to remain stationary.

EXERCISE MOVEMENT:
- Begin by bending at the knee of the attached leg and lift it towards your chest bringing the knee as close as possible to the chest.
- Continue bringing the leg up as high as you can or until you begin to feel that your supporting leg is starting to bend.
- Reverse the motion slowly back to the starting position and repeat for the scheduled number of repetitions. When finished, perform the same exercise on the supporting leg.

EXERCISE TECHNIQUE POINTS:
- Keep your abdominal muscles tensed to help prevent your pelvis from moving.
- Do not allow the supporting leg to bend at the knee as you near the top of the exercise motion.

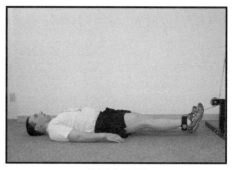
START

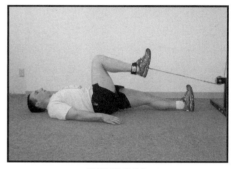
FINISH

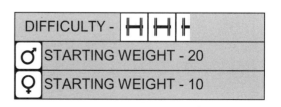

DIFFICULTY -	⊦⊣ ⊦⊣ ⊦	
♂	STARTING WEIGHT - 20	
♀	STARTING WEIGHT - 10	

FRONT THIGH AND HIP EXERCISES 59

FRONT THIGH EXERCISES

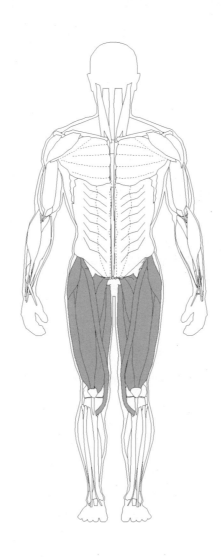

SISSY SQUATS

MAJOR MUSCLES IN USE:
   Vastus Lateralis, Rectus Femoris, Vastus Medialis

STARTING POSITION:
- While standing on your toes, place one hand waist-high on a sturdy structure (such as a bench upright). Position your feet about 8 – 10 inches apart.

EXERCISE MOVEMENT:
- Begin the movement by bending your knees. Do not bend at the waist.
- As you lower yourself, you should incline your torso backwards so that your thighs and upper body stay in a straight line.
- Your knees should lead the movement with your pelvis pushed forward as you lower yourself.
- As you lower yourself down, you should progressively lean backwards so that at the bottom of the movement your torso is about 45° to the floor.
- When you reach the bottom your calves should be touching the backs of your thighs with your heels off the floor. Now reverse the motion by straightening your legs. Your torso must stay in a straight line with your thighs.

EXERCISE TECHNIQUE POINTS:
- Do not bend at the waist.
- Stay on your toes throughout the lowering and raising portions of the movement.
- Do not bounce at the bottom.
- If necessary, you may wish to hold a barbell plate over your chest for added weight to make the exercise more difficult.

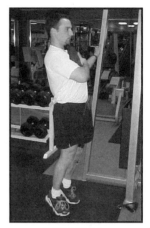

START

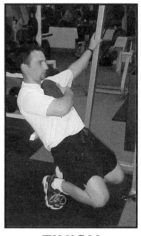

FINISH

DIFFICULTY -	H	H	H	┠
♂	STARTING WEIGHT – no weight			
♀	STARTING WEIGHT - no weight			

LEG PRESS

MAJOR MUSCLES IN USE:
Vastus Lateralis, Rectus Femoris, Vastus Medialis, Gluteus Maximus, Biceps Femoris, Semitendinosus, Semimembranosus

STARTING POSITION:
- Sit in the machine so that your lower back is pressed against the backrest.
- Place your feet about shoulder-width apart on the platform.
- Grasp the handles on either side of the seat to help brace your upper body.
- Push on the platform and release the safety catches on the leg press.

EXERCISE MOVEMENT:
- Starting with your legs extended and bent slightly at the knees, lower the platform towards you by bending your knees towards your chest.
- Keeping your heels in contact with the platform, lower the weight until your knees are just less than 90°. If your heels come off the platform before you reach 90°, try positioning your feet higher on the platform.
- Return the platform back to the starting position by straightening your legs.

EXERCISE TECHNIQUE POINTS:
- Never lock your knees.
- Do not let your lower back come off the seat.
- Make sure that your knee angle reaches at least 90°.

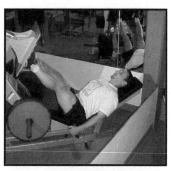

START

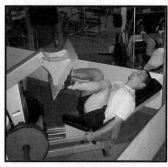

FINISH

DIFFICULTY -	⊢⊣	
♂	STARTING WEIGHT – 200	
♀	STARTING WEIGHT - 100	

ONE LEGGED PRESS

MAJOR MUSCLES IN USE:

Vastus Lateralis, Rectus Femoris, Vastus Medialis, Gluteus Maximus, Biceps Femoris, Semitendinosus, Semimembranosus

STARTING POSITION:
- Sit in the machine so that your lower back is pressed against the backrest.
- Place one foot on the platform so that your ankle, knee, and hip joints line up to make a straight line. Do not place your foot too far from or too close to the midline of your body since this will put excess force on your knee and hip.
- Grasp the handles on either side of the seat to help brace your upper body.
- Push on the platform and release the safety catches on the leg press.

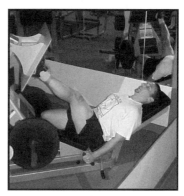

START

EXERCISE MOVEMENT:
- Starting with your leg extended but bent slightly at the knee, lower the platform towards you by bending your knee towards your chest.
- Lower the platform down until your knee angle is slightly less than 90° between your thigh and your lower leg. Your heel should remain in contact with the platform. If your heel does come off before you reach 90°, try positioning your foot higher on the platform.
- Return the platform back to the starting position by straightening your leg.

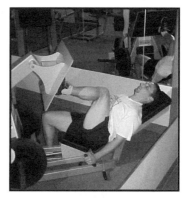

FINISH

EXERCISE TECHNIQUE POINTS:
- Never lock your knee.
- Do not let your lower back come up off the seat.
- Make sure that your knee angle reaches at least 90° or less.

DIFFICULTY -	⊢⊣ ⊢⊣	
♂	STARTING WEIGHT - 75	
♀	STARTING WEIGHT - 40	

FRONT THIGH EXERCISES 63

LEG EXTENSION

MAJOR MUSCLES IN USE:
Vastus Lateralis, Rectus Femoris, Vastus Medialis

STARTING POSITION:
- Sit on the machine so that the middle of your knee joint is lined up with the joint on the machine that is doing the movement (point of rotation).
- Your lower back should be pressed firmly against the backrest. The backs of your knees should rest against the front edge of the padded seat with your knees bent at an angle of 90° or less.
- Place the lower part of your shins behind the pad(s) on the machine.
- Grasp the handles on either side of the seat to help brace your upper body.

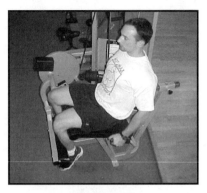

START

EXERCISE MOVEMENT:
- Using your front thigh muscles only, extend your legs, straightening the knees by kicking your feet out along the path of the machine.
- At the end of the movement your legs should be fully extended so that the knees are straight.
- Return your feet back to the starting position along the arc as you raised the weight.

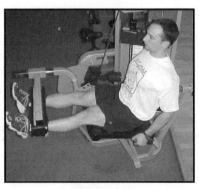

FINISH

EXERCISE TECHNIQUE POINTS:
- Do not let your buttocks come off the seat in order to help you perform the repetitions.
- Do not let your upper thighs come off the seat at the end of the motion.

DIFFICULTY -	⊦⊣	
♂	STARTING WEIGHT - 80	
♀	STARTING WEIGHT - 50	

FRONT THIGH EXERCISES

SINGLE LEG EXTENSION

MAJOR MUSCLES IN USE:
Vastus Lateralis, Rectus Femoris, Vastus Medialis

STARTING POSITION:
- Place both legs in the machine so that the backs of your knees are against the edge of the padded seat. Your knees should be bent at 90° or less.
- The leg that is being exercised should have the side of its knee joint lined up with the joint on the machine that is doing the movement (point of rotation).
- The lower portion of your shin and the front of your ankle should be placed behind the leg pad of the machine.

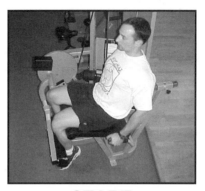

START

EXERCISE MOVEMENT:
- Using your front thigh muscles only, extend your leg at the knee by kicking your foot outwards, following the path of the machine.
- At the end of the movement your leg should be fully extended so that the knee is straight.
- Return your foot back along the same path that you raised the weight.

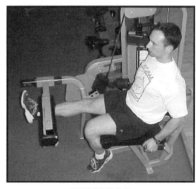

FINISH

EXERCISE TECHNIQUE POINTS:
- Do not let your buttocks come off the seat in order to help you perform the repetitions.
- Do not let your upper thigh come off the seat at the end of the motion.
- Make sure that you keep your non-exercising leg clear of the moving machinery.
- Do not allow the non-exercising leg to contribute to the motion.

DIFFICULTY -	H
♂ STARTING WEIGHT - 40	
♀ STARTING WEIGHT - 25	

FRONT THIGH EXERCISES

CABLE LEG EXTENSION

MAJOR MUSCLES IN USE:
Vastus Lateralis, Rectus Femoris, Vastus Medialis

STARTING POSITION:
- Sit on the elevated portion of an exercise bench with your back to a machine equipped with a low pulley apparatus.
- The height of the bench should be adjusted so that the foot of the leg that is being exercised does not touch the floor.
- The ankle of the exercising leg should be firmly attached to the cable with a strap.

EXERCISE MOVEMENT:
- Using your front thigh muscles only, extend your leg at the knee by kicking your foot outwards and in front of you.
- At the end of the movement your leg should be fully extended so that the knee is straight.
- Return your foot back along the same path that you raised the weight.

EXERCISE TECHNIQUE POINTS:
- Do not let your buttocks come off the seat in order to help you perform the repetitions.
- Do not let your upper thigh come off the seat at the end of the motion.
- Make sure that you keep your non-exercising leg clear of the moving machinery.
- You may wish to allow the non-exercising leg to touch the floor to help you stabilize your body.
- Keep a firm grip on the bench to help you with your balance.

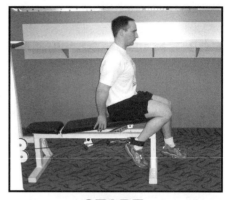

START

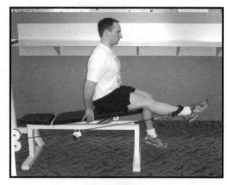

FINISH

DIFFICULTY -	H	H	H
♂	STARTING WEIGHT - 40		
♀	STARTING WEIGHT - 20		

BALL SQUATS

MAJOR MUSCLES IN USE:

Vastus Lateralis, Rectus Femoris, Vastus Medialis, Gluteus Maximus, Biceps Femoris, Semitendinosus, Semimembranosus

STARTING POSITION:
- Place an exercise ball at the midline of your body between your lower back and a flat smooth wall. Lean back against the ball by placing your feet forward so that you are leaning against the ball.
- Your feet should be shoulder-width apart with your toes pointing forward.
- Look straight ahead with your abdominal and lower back muscles tensed.
- You should position your torso with your chest up and your hands resting on your hips or holding dumbbells.

EXERCISE MOVEMENT:
- Keeping your chest up and looking straight ahead, begin to lower yourself into a squatting position by bending at the knees.
- Allow the ball to roll up your back as you lower yourself into the bottom position.
- Once your thighs are parallel to the floor, reverse the motion so that you finish in the starting position.

EXERCISE TECHNIQUE POINTS:
- Do not round your back at any time during the exercise.
- To help stabilize your balance keep your abdominal muscles tight and keep your eyes focused on an object that is stationary.

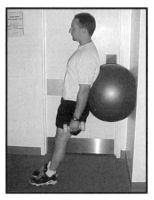

START

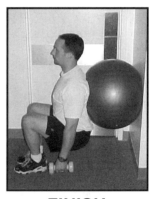

FINISH

DIFFICULTY -	�⊢ ⊢H⊢ ⊢H⊢	
♂	STARTING WEIGHT - no weight	
♀	STARTING WEIGHT - no weight	

ONE LEGGED BALL SQUATS

MAJOR MUSCLES IN USE:
Vastus Lateralis, Rectus Femoris, Vastus Medialis, Gluteus Maximus, Biceps Femoris, Semitendinosus, Semimembranosus

STARTING POSITION:
- Place an exercise ball between your lower back and a flat smooth wall. Adjust the ball so that is slightly to the side of the midline of your body nearest to the exercising leg. Lean back against the ball by placing your feet forward so that your bodyweight is shifted against the ball.
- Shift your weight onto one of your legs and cross the non-exercising leg over the front of the exercising leg.
- Look straight ahead with your abdominal and lower back muscles tensed.
- You should position your torso with your chest up and your hands on your hips or holding dumbbells.

EXERCISE MOVEMENT:
- Keeping your chest up and looking straight ahead, begin to lower yourself into a squatting position by bending at the knees.
- Allow the ball to roll up your back as you lower yourself into the bottom position.
- Once your thigh is parallel to the floor, reverse the motion so that you finish in the starting position.

EXERCISE TECHNIQUE POINTS:
- Do not round your back at any time during the exercise.
- To help with balance, keep your abdominal muscles tight and keep your eyes focused on an object that is stationary.
- You may wish to perform this exercise in a corner so that you can use the other wall to help you balance.

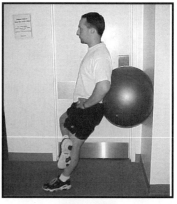

START

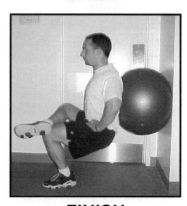

FINISH

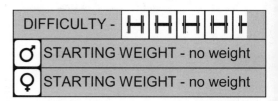

DIFFICULTY - H H H H H

♂ STARTING WEIGHT - no weight

♀ STARTING WEIGHT - no weight

FRONT THIGH EXERCISES

REAR THIGH EXERCISES

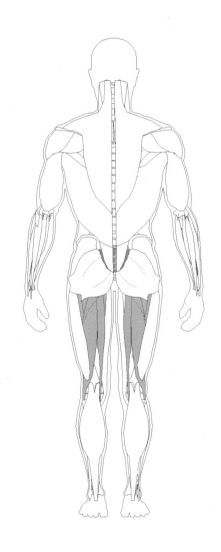

STIFF LEG DEADLIFT

MAJOR MUSCLES IN USE:
Biceps Femoris, Semitendinosus, Semimembranosus, Gluteus Maximus, Adductor Magnus, Erector Spinae

STARTING POSITION:
- Stand and hold a barbell against your upper thighs with a shoulder width, overhand or over-underhand grip.
- Feet should also be shoulder width apart.
- Knees should be slightly bent.
- Shoulders are back with your chest held high.
- Tense the abdominal and lower back muscles.

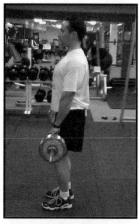

START

EXERCISE MOVEMENT:
- Slowly bend forward at the waist, allowing your hips to lead the movement by moving backwards.
- The bar should stay close to the legs as you bend forward.
- The end of the lowering portion occurs when your back is parallel to the floor and the bar is approximately at mid-shin level. At this point, reverse the movement until you are once again standing upright in the starting position.

EXERCISE TECHNIQUE POINTS:
- Make sure your back is straight by keeping your chest out and your shoulders back.
- Do not bounce in the bottom position.
- It is normal for your legs to bend slightly during the lowering portion.
- Your back should keep its normal spinal curve while you are doing the movement.
- Make sure you keep your back straight by pushing the buttocks out throughout the whole motion.

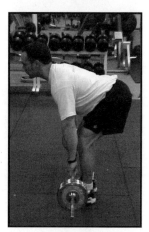

FINISH

DIFFICULTY -	H H H I⊦	
♂	STARTING WEIGHT - 65	
♀	STARTING WEIGHT - 35	

REAR THIGH EXERCISES

DUMBBELL STIFF LEG DEADLIFT

MAJOR MUSCLES IN USE:

Biceps Femoris, Semitendinosus, Semimembranosus, Gluteus Maximus, Adductor Magnus, Erector Spinae

STARTING POSITION:
- Stand and hold two dumbbells end-to-end against your upper thighs about shoulder width apart.
- Feet should be shoulder width apart.
- Knees should be slightly bent.
- Shoulders are back with your chest held high.
- Tense the abdominal and lower back muscles.

EXERCISE MOVEMENT:
- Slowly bend forward at the waist, allowing your hips to lead the movement by moving backwards.
- The dumbbells should stay close to the legs as you bend forward.
- The end of the lowering portion occurs when your back is parallel to the floor and the bars on the dumbbells are approximately at mid-shin level. At this point, reverse the movement until you are once again standing upright in the starting position.

EXERCISE TECHNIQUE POINTS:
- Make sure your back is straight by keeping your chest out and your shoulders back.
- Do not bounce in the bottom position.
- It is normal for your legs to bend slightly during the lowering portion.
- Your back should keep its normal spinal curve while you are doing the movement.
- Make sure you keep your back straight by pushing the buttocks out throughout the whole motion.

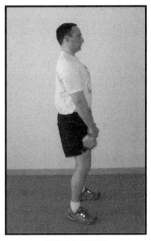

START

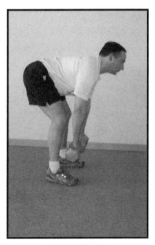

FINISH

DIFFICULTY -	H	H	H	H
♂ STARTING WEIGHT - 25				
♀ STARTING WEIGHT - 15				

REAR THIGH EXERCISES 71

CABLE STIFF LEG DEADLIFT

MAJOR MUSCLES IN USE:
Biceps Femoris, Semitendinosus, Semimembranosus, Gluteus Maximus, Adductor Magnus, Erector Spinae

STARTING POSITION:
- Stand in front of a machine equipped with a low pulley apparatus.
- Grasp a straight bar attached to the cable and hold it against your upper thighs with a shoulder width, overhand or over-underhand grip.
- Feet should also be shoulder width apart.
- Knees should be slightly bent.
- Shoulders are back with your chest held high.
- Tense the abdominal and lower back muscles.

EXERCISE MOVEMENT:
- Slowly bend forward at the waist, allowing your hips to lead the movement by moving backwards.
- As you bend forward, compensate for the pull of the cable by letting your hips push further backwards. This will shift your centre of gravity back allowing you to keep your balance.
- The end of the lowering portion occurs when your back is parallel to the floor and the bar is approximately at mid-shin level. At this point, reverse the movement until you are once again standing upright in the starting position.

EXERCISE TECHNIQUE POINTS:
- Make sure your back is straight by keeping your chest out and your shoulders back.
- Do not bounce in the bottom position.
- It is normal for your legs to bend slightly during the lowering portion.
- Your back should keep its normal spinal curve while you are doing the movement.
- Make sure you keep your back straight by pushing the buttocks out throughout the whole motion.
- You may wish to stand on a platform that is a bit higher than the pulley in order to give a farther range of motion.

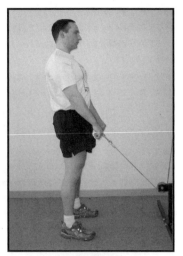

START

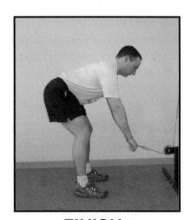

FINISH

DIFFICULTY - H H H H	
♂	STARTING WEIGHT - 70
♀	STARTING WEIGHT - 50

REAR THIGH EXERCISES

PRONE LEG CURLS

MAJOR MUSCLES IN USE:
Biceps Femoris, Semitendinosus, Semimembranosus, Gracilis

STARTING POSITION:
- Lie face down on the leg curl machine and allow your kneecaps to clear the end of the padded bench.
- Your knee joints should be lined up with the moving joint on the machine.
- The backs of your ankles should be hooked under the leg pad.
- Steady your torso by grabbing onto the handgrips attached to the machine.

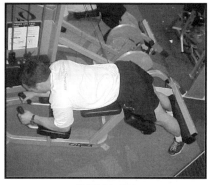

START

EXERCISE MOVEMENT:
- While keeping your upper torso stationary, bend your knees by pulling your heels up towards your hips.
- Once your knees are bent as much as possible, lower the weight back down to the starting position.

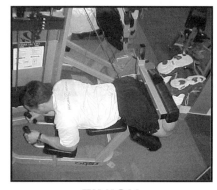

FINISH

EXERCISE TECHNIQUE POINTS:
- Do not sway your torso up and down while doing the exercise.
- It is normal for your pelvis to tilt forward as you perform the movement, but be careful to keep your hips in contact with the bench.
- Do not bounce in the bottom position.

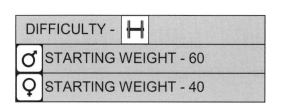

DIFFICULTY - H	
♂	STARTING WEIGHT - 60
♀	STARTING WEIGHT - 40

SINGLE PRONE LEG CURL

MAJOR MUSCLES IN USE:
Biceps Femoris, Semitendinosus, Semimembranosus, Gracilis

STARTING POSITION:
- Lie face down on the leg curl machine and allow your kneecaps to clear the padded bench.
- Your knees are to be lined up with the joint on the machine that will be moving.
- The backs of your ankles should be hooked under the leg pad.
- Steady your torso by grabbing onto the handgrips attached to the machine.

EXERCISE MOVEMENT:
- While keeping your upper torso stationary, allow only one leg to bend at the knee by bringing your heel up towards your hip.
- Once your knee is bent as much as possible, lower the weight back down to the starting position.
- Remember to keep the leg that is not lifting the weight straight.
- Once all the desired repetitions are performed for one leg, begin immediately on the opposite leg.

EXERCISE TECHNIQUE POINTS:
- Do not sway your torso up and down while doing the exercise.
- It is normal for your pelvis to tilt forward as you do the movement, but be careful to make sure that your hips stay in contact with the bench.
- Do not bounce in the bottom position.
- Keep your body as stationary as possible since the force from lifting the weight can cause your body and hips to shift position from side to side.

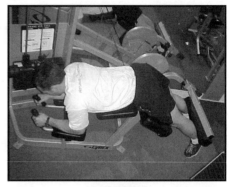

START

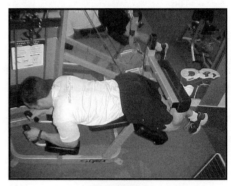

FINISH

DIFFICULTY -		
♂	STARTING WEIGHT - 30	
♀	STARTING WEIGHT - 20	

REAR THIGH EXERCISES

SEATED LEG CURL

MAJOR MUSCLES IN USE:
Biceps Femoris, Semitendinosus, Semimembranosus, Gracilis

STARTING POSITION:
- Sit in the seated leg curl machine and allow your kneecaps to just clear the padded bar that rests across the lower portion of your thighs.
- Your knee joint should be lined up with the joint on the machine that will be moving.
- The backs of your ankles should be resting on top of the leg pad and your lower back should be pushed firmly into the backrest.
- If available, attach the seat belt to secure your hips to the machine.
- Steady your torso by grabbing onto the handgrips attached to the machine.

EXERCISE MOVEMENT:
- While bracing your upper torso, bend your knees by bringing your feet down towards the floor.
- Once your knees are bent as far as possible, return the leg pad back to the starting position.

EXERCISE TECHNIQUE POINTS:
- Do not sway your torso back and forth while doing the exercise.
- Do not allow your lower back to arch excessively.
- Make sure your hips stay in contact with the backrest.

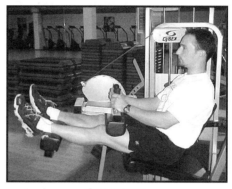

START

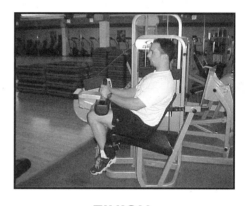

FINISH

DIFFICULTY -	⊢⊣ ⊢	
♂	STARTING WEIGHT - 65	
♀	STARTING WEIGHT - 45	

REAR THIGH EXERCISES

DUMBBELL LEG CURLS

MAJOR MUSCLES IN USE:
Biceps Femoris, Semitendinosus, Semimembranosus, Gracilis, Gastrocnemius

STARTING POSITION:
- Lie face down on a flat bench with your legs extended so that your kneecaps just clear the end of the bench.
- Bend your knees until the soles of your feet point to the ceiling. Have someone place the bar of the dumbbell between the arches of your feet. The dumbbell should be positioned so that the inside portion of the bell or plate of the dumbbell is resting flat against the bottom of your feet.
- Squeeze the bar of the dumbbell together with your feet.

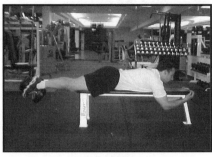
START

EXERCISE MOVEMENT:
- While keeping your upper torso stationary, slowly straighten your legs and lower the dumbbell towards the floor.
- Lower the dumbbell until your legs are almost straight.
- Before your legs become perfectly straight, immediately reverse the motion by raising the weight back up until your knees are once again bent at 90° to your body.

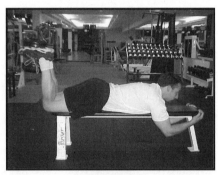
FINISH

EXERCISE TECHNIQUE POINTS:
- Do not sway your torso up and down while doing the exercise.
- It is normal for your pelvis to tilt forward as you do the movement, but avoid excessive arching of the lower back.
- Make sure your feet are always squeezed together and that your feet are pointed in the bottom position of the movement.

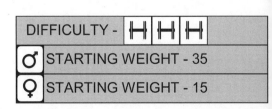

| DIFFICULTY - | ⊢⊣ ⊢⊣ ⊢⊣ |
| ♂ STARTING WEIGHT - 35 |
| ♀ STARTING WEIGHT - 15 |

STANDING CABLE LEG CURLS

MAJOR MUSCLES IN USE:
Biceps Femoris, Semitendinosus, Semimembranosus, Gracilis, Gastrocnemius

STARTING POSITION:
- Stand facing the front of a pulley machine with the cable firmly attached to the ankle of one leg while the other leg stands on a low platform.
- Position the leg on which you are standing approximately 3 – 4 feet away from the machine so that you may lean forward.
- The leg that is attached to the cable should be about 12 inches ahead of the leg you are standing on.
- Steady your upper torso by holding on to the machine. Your hips should be facing forward so that your shoulders and hips are aligned.

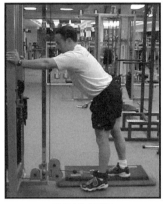

START

EXERCISE MOVEMENT:
- While keeping your upper torso stationary, bend the leg that is attached to the cable at the knee by bringing the heel up towards the buttocks.
- As you raise the weight, be careful not to allow the upper thigh to move or the hips to twist.
- Once the knee is bent as far as possible, lower the weight back to the starting position so that your leg is straight.

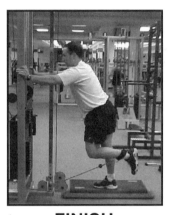

FINISH

EXERCISE TECHNIQUE POINTS:
- Do not sway your torso back and forth while doing the exercise.
- Make sure your upper thigh stays as still as possible since movement in this area will lessen the tension on the rear thigh.
- Make sure that the leg doing the exercise is clear of the floor and has a full range of motion.

DIFFICULTY -	H	H	H
♂ STARTING WEIGHT - 30			
♀ STARTING WEIGHT - 20			

REAR THIGH EXERCISES

BALL LEG CURLS

MAJOR MUSCLES IN USE:
Biceps Femoris, Semitendinosus, Semimembranosus, Gracilis, Gastrocnemius

STARTING POSITION:
- Lie on your back with your arms stretched away from your sides to help stabilize your body. Place both your feet and calves on an exercise ball.
- Lift your hips off the ground and steady yourself with your arms. Your body should be in a straight line with your feet higher than your head.

EXERCISE MOVEMENT:
- While keeping your upper body stationary, bend your legs at the knees in order to bring your heels back towards the buttocks.
- As you pull your feet towards your buttocks, keep your torso and your thighs in a straight line. As your hips rise, the ball should roll under your feet bringing your heels towards your buttocks while your toes remain on the ball.
- Return the ball back to the starting position so that your body and legs are once again in a straight line.

EXERCISE TECHNIQUE POINTS:
- Try not to let the ball move from side to side while doing the exercise.
- Make sure that your upper thighs are in a straight line with your torso and that you do not bend at the waist.
- Make sure that there are no objects or people around you that you might hit should you lose control during the exercise.
- Be certain to bring your heels back towards your buttocks as far as possible.

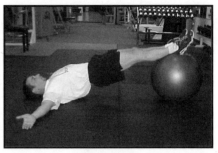
START

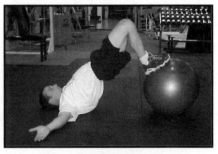
FINISH

DIFFICULTY -	⊢ ⊢ ⊢ ⊢
♂ STARTING WEIGHT - no weight	
♀ STARTING WEIGHT - no weight	

SINGLE BALL LEG CURLS

MAJOR MUSCLES IN USE:
Biceps Femoris, Semitendinosus, Semimembranosus, Gracilis, Gastrocnemius

STARTING POSITION:
- Lie on your back with your arms extended out from your shoulders to help stabilize your body (as shown in the "START" picture). Place your foot and the calf of one leg on an exercise ball. Cross the non-exercising leg across the thigh of the exercising leg.
- Lift your hips off the ground and steady yourself with your arms. Your body should be in a straight line with your feet higher than your head.

EXERCISE MOVEMENT:
- While keeping your upper torso stationary, bend your leg at the knee and bring the heel back towards the buttocks.
- As you pull your foot towards your buttocks, keep your torso and your thigh in a straight line. As your hips rise in the air, the ball should roll under your foot. Bring your heel as close to the buttocks as possible, keeping your toes on the ball.
- Return the ball back to the starting position so that your upper body is once again in a straight line with your thigh.

EXERCISE TECHNIQUE POINTS:
- Try not to let the ball move from side to side while doing the exercise.
- Make sure your upper thigh is in a straight line with your torso and you do not bend at the waist.
- Make sure that there are no objects or people near that you might hit should you lose control during the exercise.
- Be certain to bring your heel as far back towards your buttocks as possible.

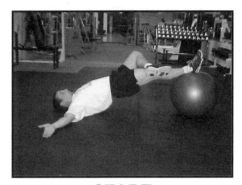

START

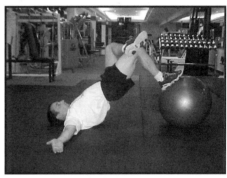

FINISH

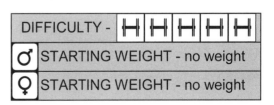

DIFFICULTY -	H	H	H	H	H
♂ STARTING WEIGHT - no weight					
♀ STARTING WEIGHT - no weight					

LYING CABLE LEG CURLS

MAJOR MUSCLES IN USE:
Biceps Femoris, Semitendinosus, Semimembranosus, Gracilis, Gastrocnemius

STARTING POSITION:
- Lie face down on a bench that is placed directly in front of the cable machine. The ankle of the leg to be exercise should be firmly attached to the lower cable. The foot of the other leg can be placed beside the former foot or on the ground beside the bench.
- Position the ankle so that it is approximately 2 – 3 feet away from the machine and directly in line with the pulley.
- Steady your body by hanging on to the bench.

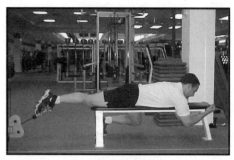

START

EXERCISE MOVEMENT:
- While keeping your torso stationary, bend the attached leg at the knee by bringing the heel up towards the buttocks.
- As you pull the weight up, be careful not to allow the upper thigh to move or the hips to twist.
- Once the knee is bent as far as possible, lower the weight back to the starting position so that your leg is once again straight.

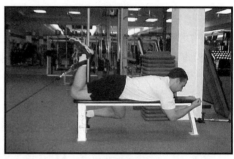

FINISH

EXERCISE TECHNIQUE POINTS:
- Do not allow your torso to lift off the bench while doing the exercise.
- Do not allow your hips to rise excessively off the bench.
- Make sure that you bend the leg along the same path as the pulley.

DIFFICULTY -	⊢	⊢
♂ STARTING WEIGHT - 25		
♀ STARTING WEIGHT - 15		

BUTTOCK EXERCISES

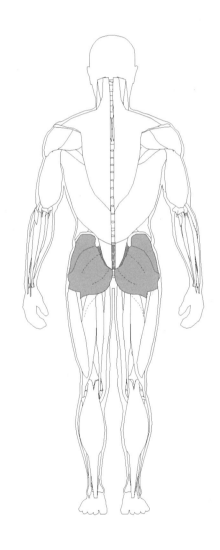

STRAIGHT LEG EXTENSIONS

MAJOR MUSCLES IN USE:
Biceps Femoris, Semitendinosus, Semimembranosus, Gluteus Maximus, Adductor Magnus, Erector Spinae

STARTING POSITION:
- Position your hips in the middle of the large pad of the hyperextension bench with your head facing the small pads and your legs positioned outwards from the machine.
- Steady your upper body by grasping the smaller pads or the frame of the machine with your hands.
- Your legs should be hanging downwards towards the floor so that your body is bent at 90°.
- Tense the abdominal and lower back muscles. You may wish to hold a dumbbell between your feet for added resistance.

EXERCISE MOVEMENT:
- Begin the movement by raising your straightened legs.
- Finish the exercise movement with your legs as high as possible.
- Lower your legs back to the starting position in the same arc that they were raised.

EXERCISE TECHNIQUE POINTS:
- Do not swing in the bottom position.
- Do not allow your legs to bend at any point in the motion.
- Your back should keep its normal spinal curves while doing the movement.
- Make sure you keep your back straight by tensing your abdominals, lower back, hamstring, and buttock muscles.

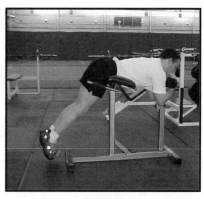

START

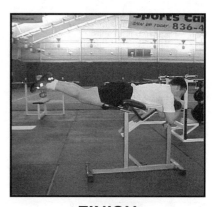

FINISH

DIFFICULTY -	H	H	H
♂ STARTING WEIGHT - no weight			
♀ STARTING WEIGHT - no weight			

BALL STRAIGHT LEG EXTENSIONS

MAJOR MUSCLES IN USE:

Biceps Femoris, Semitendinosus, Semimembranosus, Gluteus Maximus, Adductor Magnus, Erector Spinae

STARTING POSITION:

- Position your hips in the middle of an exercise ball that is balanced on the edge of an exercise bench.
- Steady your upper body by grasping on either side of the bench. Do not take your feet off the ground until you have control of your balance.
- Roll forwards slightly on the ball so that your feet are not touching the floor and your legs are hanging towards the floor. Your body should be positioned on the ball so that it is bent at 90°.
- Tense the abdominal and lower back muscles. You may wish to hold a dumbbell between your feet for added resistance.

EXERCISE MOVEMENT:

- Begin the movement by raising your straightened legs.
- Finish the exercise movement with your legs as high as possible.
- Lower your legs back to the starting position in the same arc that they were raised.

EXERCISE TECHNIQUE POINTS:

- Do not swing or bounce in the bottom position.
- Do not allow your legs to bend at any point in the motion.
- Your back should keep its normal spinal curves while doing the movement.
- Make sure you keep your back straight by tensing your abdominals, lower back, hamstring, and buttock muscles.

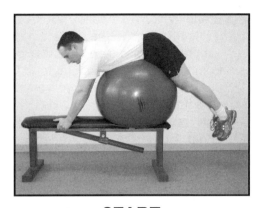

START

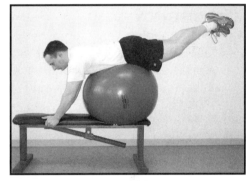

FINISH

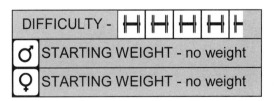

DIFFICULTY -	⊢ ⊢ ⊢ ⊢ ⊢
♂ STARTING WEIGHT - no weight	
♀ STARTING WEIGHT - no weight	

STRAIGHT LEG KICKBACK

MAJOR MUSCLES IN USE:
Biceps Femoris, Semitendinosus, Semimembranosus, Gracilis, Gastrocnemius

STARTING POSITION:
- Stand in front of a pulley machine with the cable firmly attached to the ankle of one leg while the supporting leg is standing on a low platform.
- Position the leg approximately 2 – 3 feet away from the machine so that you are standing as straight as possible.
- The leg that is attached to the cable should be about 1 foot ahead of the leg you are standing on.
- Steady your upper body by hanging on to the machine. Your hips should also be facing forward so that there is no twist in your torso or hips.

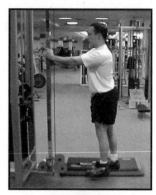

START

EXERCISE MOVEMENT:
- While keeping your upper body stationary and your attached leg as straight as possible, allow your attached leg to extend backwards by using only your buttock muscles to pull the weight back.
- As you pull the weight backwards try and stay as upright as possible in order to insure the buttock muscles do the work and not the hamstring muscles.
- Once the leg is extended as high and as far back as possible, lower the weight back to the starting position so that your exercising leg and foot are once again in front of your body.

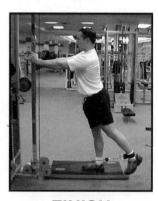

FINISH

EXERCISE TECHNIQUE POINTS:
- Do not sway your torso back and forth while doing the exercise.
- Make sure you stay as upright as possible as leaning forward will take the tension off of the buttock muscles.
- Make sure that the leg doing the exercise is locked at the knee and is clear of the floor and allows a full range of motion.

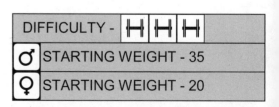

DIFFICULTY -	H H H
♂ STARTING WEIGHT - 35	
♀ STARTING WEIGHT - 20	

LOWER BODY AND BACK EXERCISES

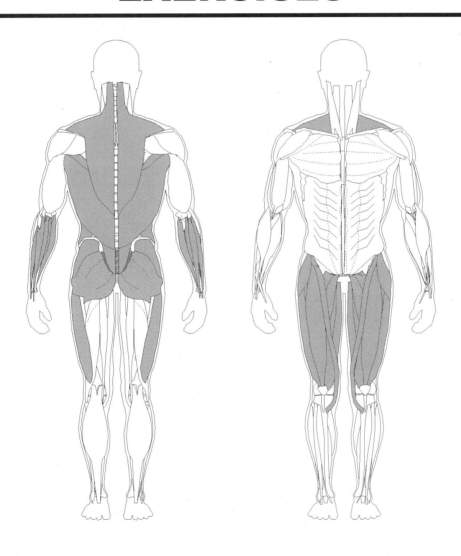

DEADLIFT

MAJOR MUSCLES IN USE:
Gluteus Maximus, Quadriceps Femoris, Trapezius, Erector Spinae, Adductor Magnus, Erector Spinae, Biceps Femoris, Semitendinosus, Semimembranosus

STARTING POSITION:
- With the barbell on the floor, stand with your feet close to the bar and positioned about shoulder width apart. Bend over and take an overhand or over-under handgrip that is a bit wider than shoulder width.
- Knees should be level or below the level of your hips.
- Shoulders are back with your chest held high so that your back is flat.
- Tense the abdominal and lower back muscles.

EXERCISE MOVEMENT:
- Begin the movement by straightening your legs until the bar reaches about knee level. From this point extend your torso by standing straight up while continuing to lift with the legs.
- Continue to raise the bar until you are standing straight up finishing with the bar at about mid-thigh level.
- Reverse the movement by lowering the bar in the opposite movement that you lifted it.

EXERCISE TECHNIQUE POINTS:
- Make sure your back is always straight with a slight arch in the lower back.
- Do not bend your arms at any point in the motion.
- Keep the bar close to your legs at all times.
- Keep your hips low at the start of the motion.

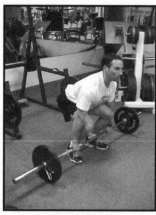

START

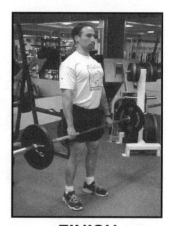

FINISH

DIFFICULTY -	H H H	
♂	STARTING WEIGHT - 95	
♀	STARTING WEIGHT - 55	

SUMO DEADLIFT

MAJOR MUSCLES IN USE:
Gluteus Maximus, Quadriceps Femoris, Trapezius, Erector Spinae, Adductor Magnus, Erector Spinae, Biceps Femoris, Semitendinosus, Semimembranosus

STARTING POSITION:
- With the barbell on the floor, stand with your feet much wider than shoulder width and your legs positioned close to the bar. Bend over and take an overhand or over-underhand grip on the bar so that your hands are about 12 to 16 inches apart.
- Knees should be level with or below the level of your hips.
- Keep your shoulders back with your chest held high so that your back is flat.
- Tense the abdominal and lower back muscles.

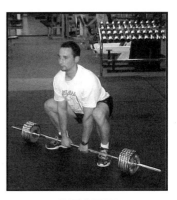

START

EXERCISE MOVEMENT:
- Begin the movement by straightening your legs until the bar reaches about knee level. From this point, extend your torso by standing straight up while continuing to lift with the legs.
- Continue to raise the bar until you are standing straight up with the bar about mid-thigh level.
- Reverse the movement by lowering the bar in the opposite movement that you lifted it.

EXERCISE TECHNIQUE POINTS:
- Make sure your back is always straight with a slight arch in the lower back by keeping your chest out and your shoulders back.
- Do not bend your arms at any point in the motion.
- Keep the bar close to your legs at all times.
- Do not allow your hips to rise too high at the start of the motion.

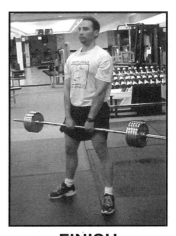

FINISH

DIFFICULTY -	H H H
♂ STARTING WEIGHT - 95	
♀ STARTING WEIGHT - 55	

UPPER BODY EXERCISES

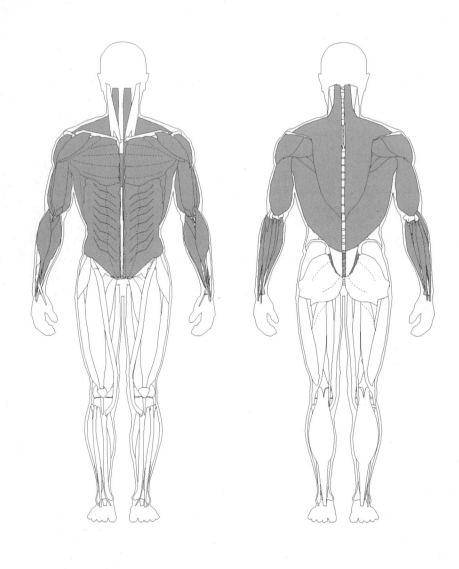

CLEANS

MAJOR MUSCLES IN USE:
Gluteus Maximus, Quadriceps Femoris, Trapezius, Erector Spinae, Adductor Magnus, Biceps Femoris, Semitendinosus, Semimembranosus

STARTING POSITION:
- With the barbell on the floor, stand with your feet about shoulder-width apart and your legs close to the bar. Bend over and take an overhand or over-underhand grip a little wider than shoulder-width.
- Knees should be level with or below the level of your hips.
- Shoulders are held back with your chest high so that your back is flat.
- Tense the abdominal and lower back muscles.

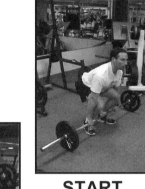

START

EXERCISE MOVEMENT:
- Begin the movement by rapidly straightening your legs until the bar reaches about knee level. From this point extend your torso as rapidly as possible by standing up while continuing to lift with the legs.
- Continue to raise the bar using the momentum generated from the first part of the lift until the bar reaches chest level. Dip your body down about 6 inches and snap your elbows under the bar to support the bar at shoulder level.
- Reverse the movement by lowering the bar in the opposite movement that you had lifted it.

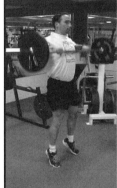

MIDDLE

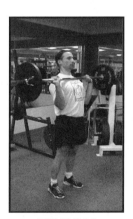

FINISH

EXERCISE TECHNIQUE POINTS:
- Make sure your back is always straight with a slight arch in the lower back by keeping your chest out and your shoulders back.
- Perform the lifting motion as quickly as possible in order to generate enough momentum to lift the bar at the end of the movement.
- Keep the bar close to your body at all times.
- Do not allow your hips to rise too high at the start of the motion.

DIFFICULTY -	⊢ ⊢ ⊢ ⊢
♂	STARTING WEIGHT - 65
♀	STARTING WEIGHT - 40

CLEAN AND PRESS

MAJOR MUSCLES IN USE:

Gluteus Maximus, Quadriceps Femoris, Trapezius, Erector Spinae, Adductor Magnus, Biceps Femoris, Semitendinosus, Semimembranosus, Anterior Deltoid, Lateral Deltoid

STARTING POSITION:
- With the barbell on the floor, stand with your feet about shoulder-width apart and your legs close to the bar. Bend over and take an overhand or over-underhand grip a little wider than shoulder-width.
- Knees should be level with or below the level of your hips.
- Shoulders are held back with your chest high so that your back is flat.
- Tense the abdominal and lower back muscles.

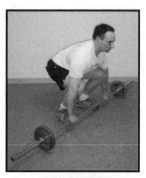

START

EXERCISE MOVEMENT:
- Begin the movement by rapidly straightening your legs until the bar reaches about knee level. From this point extend your torso as rapidly as possible by standing up while continuing to lift with the legs.
- Continue to raise the bar using the momentum generated from the first part of the lift until the bar reaches chest level. Dip your body down about 6 inches and snap your elbows under the bar to support the bar at shoulder level.
- Continue the movement by bending the knees and rapidly straightening them in order to gain enough momentum to begin pushing the barbell up. Continue to push the barbell up until your arms are fully extended and your elbows are almost locked.
- Reverse the movement by lowering the bar carefully back to the starting position.

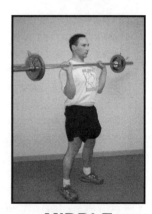

MIDDLE

EXERCISE TECHNIQUE POINTS:
- Make sure your back is always straight with a slight arch in the lower back by keeping your chest out and your shoulders back.
- Perform the lifting motion as quickly as possible in order to generate enough momentum to lift the bar at the end of the movement.
- Keep the bar close to your body at all times.
- Do not allow your hips to rise too high at the start of the motion.
- Always keep your abdominal and lower back muscles tensed throughout the whole exercise.

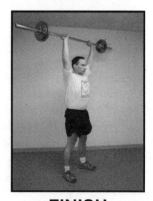

FINISH

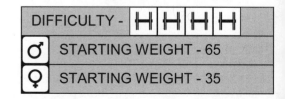

DIFFICULTY -	H H H H
♂	STARTING WEIGHT - 65
♀	STARTING WEIGHT - 35

DUMBBELL CLEANS

MAJOR MUSCLES IN USE:
Gluteus Maximus, Quadriceps Femoris, Trapezius, Erector Spinae, Adductor Magnus, Biceps Femoris, Semitendinosus, Semimembranosus

STARTING POSITION:
- With two dumbbells placed on the floor, stand with your feet about shoulder-width apart and your legs close to the dumbbells. Bend over and take an overhand grip and place your hands slightly wider than shoulder width.
- Knees should be level with or below the level of your hips.
- Shoulders are held back with your chest high so that your back is flat.
- Tense the abdominal and lower back muscles.

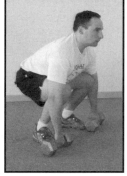

START

EXERCISE MOVEMENT:
- Begin the movement by rapidly straightening your legs until the dumbbells reach about knee level. From this point extend your torso as rapidly as possible by standing up while continuing to lift with the legs.
- Continue to raise the dumbbells, with your palms facing the floor, using the momentum generated from the first part of the lift until the dumbbells reach chest level. Dip your body down about 6 inches and snap your elbows under the dumbbells to support them at shoulder level.
- Reverse the movement by lowering the dumbbells in the opposite movement that you had lifted them.

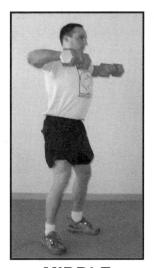

MIDDLE

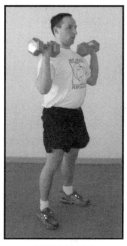

FINISH

EXERCISE TECHNIQUE POINTS:
- Make sure your back is always straight with a slight arch in the lower back by keeping your chest out and your shoulders back.
- Perform the lifting motion as quickly as possible in order to generate enough momentum to lift the dumbbells at the end of the movement.
- Keep the dumbbells close to your body at all times.
- Do not allow your hips to rise too high at the start of the motion.
- Make sure that the palms of your hands are always facing downwards during the lifting portion of the movement.
- Try to keep the dumbbells the same distance apart throughout the movement.

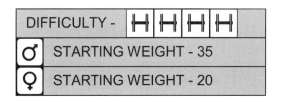

DIFFICULTY -	H H H H
♂	STARTING WEIGHT - 35
♀	STARTING WEIGHT - 20

DUMBBELL CLEAN AND PRESS

MAJOR MUSCLES IN USE:

Gluteus Maximus, Quadriceps Femoris, Trapezius, Erector Spinae, Adductor Magnus, Biceps Femoris, Semitendinosus, Semimembranosus

STARTING POSITION:

- With two dumbbells placed on the floor, stand with your feet about shoulder-width apart and your legs close to the dumbbells. Bend over and take an overhand grip and place your hands slightly wider than shoulder width.
- Knees should be level with or below the level of your hips. Shoulders are held back with your chest high so that your back is flat.
- Tense the abdominal and lower back muscles.

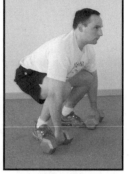

START

EXERCISE MOVEMENT:

- Begin the movement by rapidly straightening your legs until the dumbbells reach about knee level. From this point extend your torso as rapidly as possible by standing up while continuing to lift with the legs.
- Using the momentum generated from the first part of the motion, continue to lift the dumbbells to chest level. Dip your body down about 6 inches and snap your elbows under the dumbbells to support them at shoulder level.
- Continue the movement by bending the knees and rapidly straightening them in order to gain enough momentum to begin pushing the dumbbells up. Continue to push the dumbbells up until your arms are fully extended and your elbows are almost locked.
- Reverse the movement by lowering the dumbbells in the opposite movement that you had lifted them.

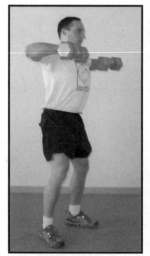

MIDDLE

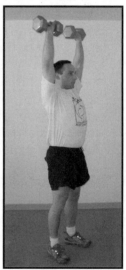

FINISH

EXERCISE TECHNIQUE POINTS:

- Your back must always be straight with a slight arch in the lower back.
- Perform the lifting motion explosively in order to generate enough momentum.
- Keep the dumbbells close to your body.
- Do not allow your hips to rise too high at the start of the motion.
- Make sure that the palms of your hands are always facing downwards during the lifting portion of the movement.
- Try to keep the dumbbells the same distance apart throughout the movement.

DIFFICULTY -	H H H H
♂	STARTING WEIGHT - 25
♀	STARTING WEIGHT - 15

UPPER BODY EXERCISES

HANG CLEANS

MAJOR MUSCLES IN USE:
Trapezius, Erector Spinae, Biceps Brachii, Deltoids

STARTING POSITION:
- Standing with your legs straight and feet about shoulder width apart.
- Arms should hang straight at your sides with the bar resting on your upper thighs.
- Take an overhand grip with hands about shoulder-width apart on the bar.

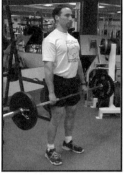

START

EXERCISE MOVEMENT:
- Begin the movement by rising up on your toes a few inches in order to help lift the weight and generate enough momentum to raise the weight to shoulder level.
- As the bar approaches shoulder level, dip your body down and snap your elbows under the bar to support the bar at shoulder level.
- Reverse the movement by lowering the bar in the opposite direction that you lifted it.

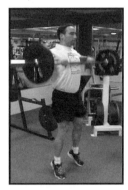

MIDDLE

EXERCISE TECHNIQUE POINTS
- Make sure your back is always straight with a slight arch in the lower back by keeping your chest up and your shoulders back.
- Perform the lifting motion as quickly as possible in order to generate enough momentum to lift the bar at the end of the movement.
- Keep the bar close to your body at all times.

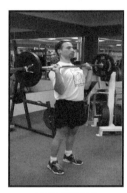

FINISH

DIFFICULTY -	H H H H	
♂	STARTING WEIGHT - 65	
♀	STARTING WEIGHT - 35	

HANG CLEAN AND PRESS

MAJOR MUSCLES IN USE:
Trapezius, Erector Spinae, Biceps Brachii, Triceps Brachii, Deltoids

STARTING POSITION:
- Standing with your legs straight and feet about shoulder width apart.
- Arms should hang straight at your sides with the bar resting on your upper thighs.
- Take an overhand grip with hands about shoulder-width apart on the bar.

EXERCISE MOVEMENT:
- Begin the movement by rising up on your toes a few inches in order to help lift the weight and generate enough momentum to raise the weight to shoulder level.
- As the bar approaches shoulder level, dip your body down and snap your elbows under the bar to support the bar at shoulder level.
- Continue the movement by bending the knees and rapidly straightening them in order to gain enough momentum to begin pushing the barbell up. Continue to push the barbell up until your arms are fully extended and your elbows are almost locked.
- Reverse the movement by lowering the bar in the opposite direction that you lifted it.

EXERCISE TECHNIQUE POINTS:
- Make sure your back is always straight with a slight arch in the lower back by keeping your chest up and your shoulders back.
- Perform the lifting motion as quickly as possible in order to generate enough momentum to lift the bar at the end of the movement.
- Keep the bar close to your body at all times.
- Always keep your abdominal and lower back muscles tensed throughout the whole exercise.

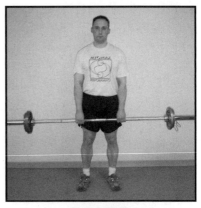

START

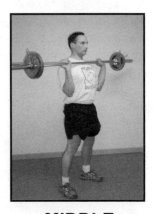

MIDDLE

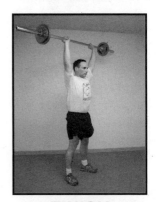

FINISH

DIFFICULTY -	H H H H
♂	STARTING WEIGHT - 40
♀	STARTING WEIGHT - 20

UPPER BODY EXERCISES

SLOW CLEAN AND PRESS

MAJOR MUSCLES IN USE:
Trapezius, Erector Spinae, Biceps Brachii, Triceps Brachii, Deltoids

STARTING POSITION:
- Standing with your legs straight and feet about shoulder width apart.
- Arms should hang straight at your sides with the bar resting on your upper thighs.
- Take an overhand grip with hands about shoulder-width apart on the bar.

EXERCISE MOVEMENT:
- Begin the movement by pulling the bar up towards your collarbone, allowing your elbows to move upwards and outwards.
- As the bar approaches shoulder level, rotate the bar towards your body by allowing your elbows to drop below the level of the bar and under your wrists.
- Continue the movement by pushing the barbell up over your head until your arms are fully extended and your elbows are almost locked.
- Reverse the movement by lowering the bar in the opposite direction that you lifted it.

EXERCISE TECHNIQUE POINTS:
- Make sure your back is always straight with a slight arch in the lower back by keeping your chest up and your shoulders back.
- Perform the lifting motion as smoothly as possible with minimal pauses.
- Try to lift the bar to collarbone level before attempting to rotate it and positioning your elbows under your wrists.
- Keep the bar close to your body at all times.
- Always keep your abdominal and lower back muscles tensed throughout the whole exercise.

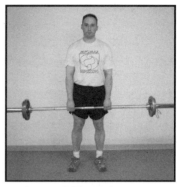

START

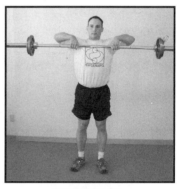

MIDDLE

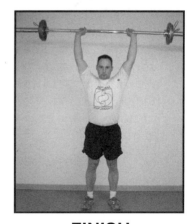

FINISH

DIFFICULTY -	H	H	H	H
♂ STARTING WEIGHT - 45				
♀ STARTING WEIGHT - 25				

DUMBBELL HANG CLEANS

MAJOR MUSCLES IN USE:
Trapezius, Erector Spinae, Biceps Brachii, Deltoids

STARTING POSITION:
- Standing with your legs straight and feet about shoulder width apart.
- Arms should hang straight at your sides with the dumbbells at the level of your upper thighs.
- Take an overhand grip with hands about shoulder-width apart.

EXERCISE MOVEMENT:
- Begin the movement by rising up on your toes a few inches in order to help lift the weight and generate enough momentum to raise the weight to shoulder level.
- As the bar approaches shoulder level, dip your body down and snap your elbows under the dumbbells to support them at shoulder level.
- Reverse the movement by lowering the dumbbells in the opposite direction that you lifted them.

EXERCISE TECHNIQUE POINTS:
- Make sure your back is always straight with a slight arch in the lower back by keeping your chest up and your shoulders back.
- Perform the lifting motion as quickly as possible in order to generate enough momentum to lift the bar at the end of the movement.
- Keep the bar close to your body at all times.
- Make sure that the palms of your hands are always facing downwards during the lifting portion of the movement.
- Try to keep the dumbbells the same distance apart throughout the movement.

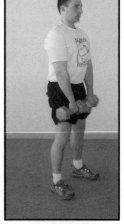

START

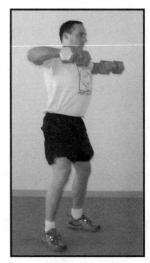

MIDDLE

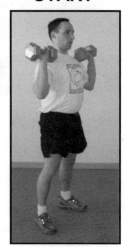

FINISH

DIFFICULTY -	H H H H
♂	STARTING WEIGHT - 30
♀	STARTING WEIGHT - 20

UPPER BODY EXERCISES

DUMBBELL HANG CLEAN AND PRESS

MAJOR MUSCLES IN USE:
Trapezius, Erector Spinae, Biceps Brachii, Deltoids

STARTING POSITION:
- Standing with your legs straight and feet about shoulder width apart.
- Arms should hang straight at your sides with the dumbbells at the level of your upper thighs.
- Take an overhand grip with hands about shoulder-width apart.

EXERCISE MOVEMENT:
- Begin the movement by rising up on your toes a few inches in order to help lift the weight and generate enough momentum to raise the weight to shoulder level.
- As the bar approaches shoulder level, dip your body down and snap your elbows under the dumbbells to support them at shoulder level.
- Continue the movement by bending the knees and rapidly straightening them in order to gain enough momentum to begin pushing the dumbbells up. Continue to push the dumbbells up until your arms are fully extended and your elbows are almost locked.
- Reverse the movement by lowering the dumbbells in the opposite direction that you lifted them.

EXERCISE TECHNIQUE POINTS:
- Make sure your back is always straight with a slight arch in the lower back by keeping your chest up and your shoulders back.
- Perform the lifting motion as quickly as possible in order to generate enough momentum to lift the bar at the end of the movement.
- Keep the bar close to your body at all times.
- Make sure that the palms of your hands are always facing downwards during the lifting portion of the movement.
- Try to keep the dumbbells the same distance apart throughout the movement.
- Always keep your abdominal and lower back muscles tensed throughout the whole exercise.

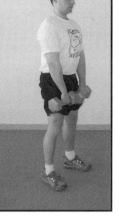

START

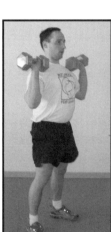

MIDDLE

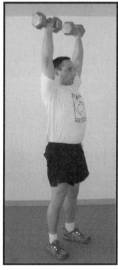

FINISH

DIFFICULTY -	H H H H	
♂	STARTING WEIGHT - 25	
♀	STARTING WEIGHT - 15	

SLOW DUMBBELL CLEAN AND PRESS

MAJOR MUSCLES IN USE:
Trapezius, Erector Spinae, Biceps Brachii, Deltoids

STARTING POSITION:
- Standing with your legs straight and feet about shoulder width apart.
- Arms should hang straight at your sides with the dumbbells at the level of your upper thighs.
- Take an overhand grip with hands about shoulder-width apart.

EXERCISE MOVEMENT:
- Begin the movement by pulling the dumbbells up towards your collarbone, allowing your elbows to move upwards and outwards. The dumbbells should travel along the path of a narrow letter "V"
- As the dumbbells approach shoulder level, rotate the dumbbells towards your body by allowing your elbows to drop below the level of the bars and directly under your wrists.
- Continue the movement by pushing the dumbbells up over your head until your arms are fully extended and your elbows are almost locked.
- Reverse the movement by lowering the weights in the opposite direction that you lifted them.

EXERCISE TECHNIQUE POINTS:
- Make sure your back is always straight with a slight arch in the lower back by keeping your chest up and your shoulders back.
- Keep the bar close to your body at all times.
- Make sure that the palms of your hands are always facing downwards during the lifting portion of the movement.
- Try not to let the dumbbells twist as you rotate them into the pressing phase of the exercise.
- Always keep your abdominal and lower back muscles tensed throughout the whole exercise.

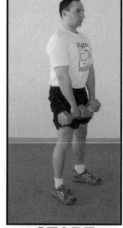

START

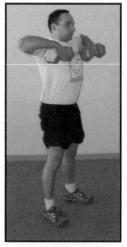

MIDDLE

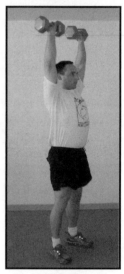

FINISH

DIFFICULTY -	H H H H	
♂	STARTING WEIGHT - 25	
♀	STARTING WEIGHT - 15	

UPPER BODY EXERCISES

DUMBBELL PULLOVER

MAJOR MUSCLES IN USE:
Latissimus Dorsi, Triceps Brachii, Pectoralis Major, Serratus Anterior

STARTING POSITION:
- Lie flat on your back and position your body across an exercise bench.
- Hold a dumbbell above your chest with your arms just slightly bent at the elbows.
- Hold the dumbbell by cupping your hand around the inside of the bell.

EXERCISE MOVEMENT:
- While keeping your elbows locked in a slightly bent position, lower the dumbbell down so that it travels along a semi-circular path towards the floor. The dumbbell should travel over your head and away from your body.
- Lower the bar down as far as possible and then raise it back to the starting position along the same path that it was lowered.

EXERCISE TECHNIQUE POINTS:
- Keep your body as still as possible and try not to arch your lower back or let your feet lose contact with the ground.
- Try to keep your elbows the same distance apart as when you started the exercise.
- Make sure your elbows are always slightly bent in order to focus more on the upper body muscles.
- As your lower the dumbbell you may wish to drop your hips lower than the level of the bench in order to stop yourself from being pulled over the bench.

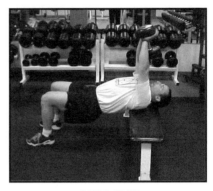

START

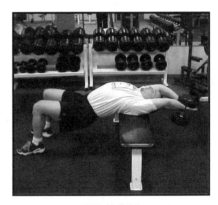

FINISH

DIFFICULTY -	⫟ ⫟ ⫟	
♂	STARTING WEIGHT - 20	
♀	STARTING WEIGHT - 10	

UPPER BODY EXERCISES 99

BACK EXERCISES

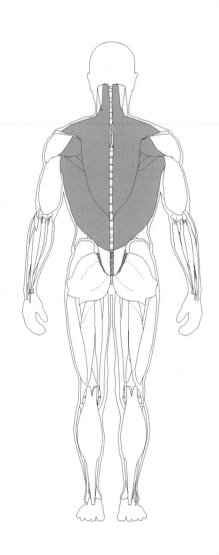

WIDE GRIP LAT PULLDOWNS TO THE FRONT

MAJOR MUSCLES IN USE:
Latissimus Dorsi, Teres major, Biceps Brachii, Brachialis, Posterior Deltoid

STARTING POSITION:
- Sit at a pulldown machine with a long bar handle attached, place your knees under the knee pad and take an overhand grip 6 - 8 inches wider than shoulder-width.
- Begin with your arms straight and your chest held high. Lean back slightly so that there is a slight arch in your upper back.

EXERCISE MOVEMENT:
- While keeping your elbows held back and a slight arch in your back, pull the bar down to touch your upper chest or collarbone.
- Return the bar to the starting position at a moderate pace. When finished your arms should once again be straight.

EXERCISE TECHNIQUE POINTS:
- Do not round your back by allowing your chest to lower while pulling down.
- Do not lean back excessively or rock back and forth in order to complete the repetitions.
- Always make sure your elbows are pointing to the back.

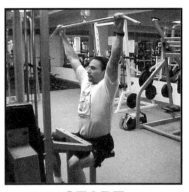

START

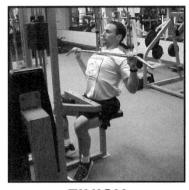

FINISH

DIFFICULTY - ⊢⊢ ⊢⊢	
♂	STARTING WEIGHT - 70
♀	STARTING WEIGHT - 45

WIDE GRIP LAT PULLDOWNS TO THE BACK

MAJOR MUSCLES IN USE:
Latissimus Dorsi, Teres major, Trapezius (lower portion), Biceps Brachii, Brachialis

STARTING POSITION:
- Sitting at the Pulldown machine with the long bar attached to the cable and your knees under the knee pad, take an overhand grip 8 - 12 inches wider than shoulder width.
- Begin with arms straight, your chest up, and leaning slightly forward while keeping a slight arch in your upper back.

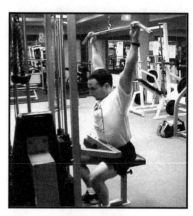

START

EXERCISE MOVEMENT:
- While keeping your elbows back and with an arch in your upper back, pull the bar down behind the head just to the base of the neck. Depending on your flexibility you may only be able to reach the base of your skull.
- At the bottom portion of the movement your elbows should be pointing slightly backwards with your shoulder blades squeezed together.
- Return the bar to the starting position at a moderate pace. When finished your arms should be straight.

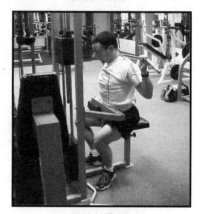

FINISH

EXERCISE TECHNIQUE POINTS:
- Do not round your back by allowing your chest to lower while pulling down.
- Do not lean excessively forward or rock back and forth in order to complete the repetitions.
- Always make sure your elbows are pointing back at the end of the movement.
- Be careful not to allow your arms to rotate excessively as this can increase your risk of injury.

DIFFICULTY - H H	
♂	STARTING WEIGHT - 60
♀	STARTING WEIGHT - 40

CLOSE GRIP PULLDOWNS

MAJOR MUSCLES IN USE:
Latissimus Dorsi, Teres Major, Biceps Brachii, Brachialis

STARTING POSITION:
- Sitting at the Pulldown machine with the Close Grip handle attached to the cable, place your knees under the kneepad and take an overhand grip with your palms facing each other.
- Begin with arms straight, lean back slightly while a keeping an arch in your upper back.

EXERCISE MOVEMENT:
- While keeping your elbows tucked in, arch your back by raising your chest and pull the handle down close to your upper chest.
- Return the bar to the starting position at a moderate pace. When finished your arms should once again be straight.

EXERCISE TECHNIQUE POINTS:
- Do not round your back by allowing your chest to lower while pulling down.
- Do not lean back excessively or rock back and forth in order to complete the repetitions.
- Always make sure your elbows are pointing back and are tucked in close to your body.

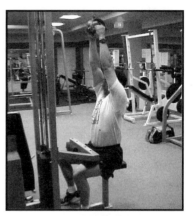

START

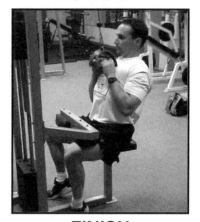

FINISH

DIFFICULTY -	⊢	⊢
♂ STARTING WEIGHT - 80		
♀ STARTING WEIGHT - 50		

NARROW GRIP PULLDOWNS

MAJOR MUSCLES IN USE:
Latissimus Dorsi, Teres Major, Biceps Brachii, Brachialis

STARTING POSITION:
- Sit at the Pulldown machine with your knees under the kneepad. Attach the long bar handle and take an overhand grip with hands just less than shoulder width apart.
- Begin with your arms straight and your chest up, lean back slightly, and maintain a small arch in your upper back.

EXERCISE MOVEMENT:
- While keeping the arch in your upper back, pull the bar down to touch your upper chest or collarbone.
- Return the bar to the starting position at a moderate pace. When finished your arms should be straight.

EXERCISE TECHNIQUE POINTS:
- Do not round your back by allowing your chest to lower while pulling down.
- Do not lean excessively back or rock back and forth in order to complete the repetitions.
- Always make sure your elbows are pointing back at the end of the movement.

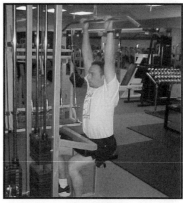

START

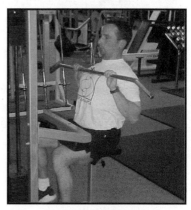

FINISH

DIFFICULTY -	⊢	⊢
♂ STARTING WEIGHT - 80		
♀ STARTING WEIGHT - 50		

BACK EXERCISES

PARALLEL GRIP PULLDOWNS

MAJOR MUSCLES IN USE:
Latissimus Dorsi, Teres Major, Biceps Brachli, Brachialis

STARTING POSITION:
- Sit at the Pulldown machine with the parallel bar handle attached to the cable. Place your knees under the kneepad and take an overhand grip on the bar with your palms facing each other.
- Begin with your arms straight, chest up, and leaning back slightly with a small arch in your upper back.

EXERCISE MOVEMENT:
- While keeping your elbows facing outwards, arch your upper back by raising your chest. Lean back and pull the bar down so that it touches between your collarbone and upper chest.
- Return the bar to the starting position at a moderate pace. When finished your arms should be straight.

EXERCISE TECHNIQUE POINTS:
- Do not round your back by lowering your chest while pulling the bar down.
- Do not lean excessively back or rock back and forth in order to complete the repetitions.
- Always make sure your elbows are pointing down and slightly to the back at the end of the exercise movement.

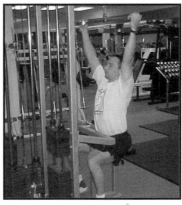

START

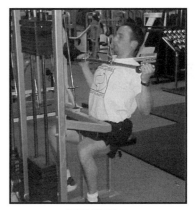

FINISH

DIFFICULTY -	⊢ ⊢	
♂	STARTING WEIGHT - 70	
♀	STARTING WEIGHT - 40	

ONE ARM LAT PULLDOWN

MAJOR MUSCLES IN USE:
Latissimus Dorsi, Teres Major, Biceps Brachii, Brachialis

STARTING POSITION:
- Sit at the Pulldown machine with your knees under the kneepad. Take an overhand grip on a single handle; your palm should be facing forward.
- Begin with your arm straight. Lean back slightly and keep your chest up.

EXERCISE MOVEMENT:
- Arch your back by raising your chest and pull the handle down close to your upper chest. Keep your elbows close to your torso.
- Return the bar to the starting position at a moderate pace. When finished your arm should be straight.

EXERCISE TECHNIQUE POINTS:
- Do not round your back by allowing your chest to lower while pulling down.
- Do not lean too far back or sway back and forth in order to complete the repetitions.
- Always make sure your elbow is tucked in close to your body.

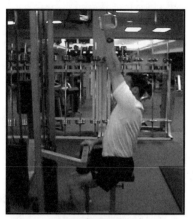

START

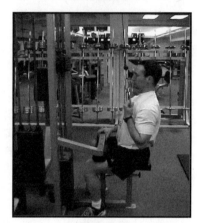

FINISH

DIFFICULTY -	H H H
♂ STARTING WEIGHT - 40	
♀ STARTING WEIGHT - 20	

REVERSE GRIP LAT PULLDOWNS

MAJOR MUSCLES IN USE:
Latissimus Dorsi, Teres Major, Trapezius (lower portion), Biceps Brachii, Brachialis

STARTING POSITION:
- Sit at the Pulldown machine with your knees under the kneepads. Attach the long bar handle and take an underhand grip so that your hands are right in front of your shoulders.
- Begin with your arms straight, chest up, and lean back slightly.

EXERCISE MOVEMENT:
- While keeping your chest high, pull the bar down in front of you so that the bar touches middle of your chest.
- At the bottom portion of the movement your elbows should be pointing to the back so that your upper arms are pulled back as far as possible.
- Return the bar to the starting position at a moderate pace. When finished your arms should be straight.

EXERCISE TECHNIQUE POINTS:
- Do not round your back by allowing your chest to lower while pulling down.
- Do not lean excessively back or rock back and forth in order to complete the repetitions.
- Make sure your hands are no farther than shoulder-width apart.

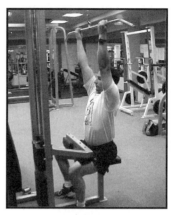

START

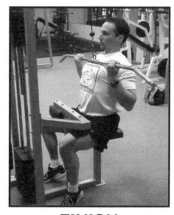

FINISH

DIFFICULTY -	⊢⊣ ⊢⊣	
♂	STARTING WEIGHT - 80	
♀	STARTING WEIGHT - 50	

BACK EXERCISES

CABLE CROSS-OVER PULLDOWNS

MAJOR MUSCLES IN USE:
Latissimus Dorsi, Teres Major, Biceps Brachii, Brachialis, Posterior Deltoid

STARTING POSITION:
- Kneel between the two high pulleys of a cable cross-over machine.
- Grasp each handle with the opposite hand to the pulley (right hand grasps the handle on the left, left hand grasps the handle to your right) and allow your hands to cross above your head with your arms extended.
- Your arms should be slightly bent at the elbows with your elbows pointing outwards and the palms of your hands facing forwards.

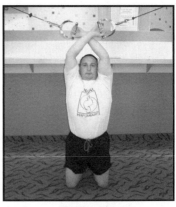

START

EXERCISE MOVEMENT:
- Keeping your elbows pointed to the side and your chest held high with a slight arch in your back, pull the handles downwards and out to the sides of your shoulders in a semicircular motion.
- Return the handles to the starting position at a moderate pace. When finished your arms should once again be crossed at your wrists.

EXERCISE TECHNIQUE POINTS:
- Do not round your back by allowing your chest to lower while pulling down.
- Do not lean back excessively or rock back and forth in order to complete the repetitions.
- Always make sure your elbows are pointing to the side and slightly back.
- You may find it easier to control the motion if you sit on your feet while kneeling.

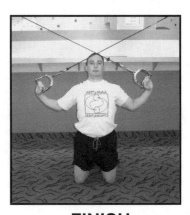

FINISH

DIFFICULTY -	H H H H
♂ STARTING WEIGHT - 30	
♀ STARTING WEIGHT - 15	

WIDE GRIP PULL-UPS (CHINS) TO THE FRONT

MAJOR MUSCLES IN USE:
Latissimus Dorsi, Teres Major, Biceps Brachii, Brachialis

STARTING POSITION:
- Standing at the chin-up bar, take an overhand grip about 6 - 8 inches wider than shoulder-width.
- While hanging with your arms straight, stabilize your shoulders by tensing the back and shoulder muscles.

EXERCISE MOVEMENT:
- As you pull yourself up, raise your chest and lean back slightly to allow the back muscle to do the majority of the lifting.
- Try to touch your upper chest to the bar. If this is not possible, you should be able to lift yourself high enough so that you chin is level with the bar.
- Lower yourself back to the starting position so that your arms are fully extended.

EXERCISE TECHNIQUE POINTS:
- Do not round your back by allowing your chest to lower while pulling up.
- Pull yourself up smoothly without any jerking or kicking movements.
- Make sure your arms are fully extended at the bottom. If you cannot pull yourself up from a fully extended position or you cannot pull yourself high enough, you are not strong enough to do this exercise on your own yet. You may need the help of a spotter.

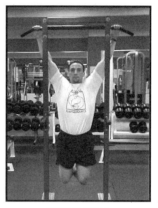

START

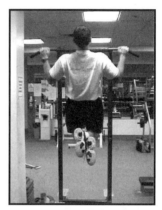

FINISH

DIFFICULTY -	H	H
♂ STARTING WEIGHT - no weight		
♀ STARTING WEIGHT - no weight		

WIDE GRIP PULL-UPS (CHINS) TO THE BACK

MAJOR MUSCLES IN USE:
Latissimus Dorsi, Teres Major, Biceps Brachii, Brachialis

STARTING POSITION:
- Standing at a long chin-up bar, take an overhand grip 8 - 12 inches wider than shoulder width.
- While hanging with your arms straight, stabilize your shoulders by tensing the shoulder and back muscles.

EXERCISE MOVEMENT:
- As you pull yourself up, lean forward by bringing your knees backwards. This will cause your torso to lean forward.
- Try to touch the base of the back of your neck to the bar. If this is not possible, you should be able to lift yourself high enough so that the middle of the back of your head is level with the bar.
- Lower yourself back to the starting position so that your arms are fully extended.

EXERCISE TECHNIQUE POINTS:
- Make sure you pull yourself up smoothly without any jerking or kicking movements.
- Your elbows should be pointing backwards once you reach the top of the movement.
- Make sure your arms are fully extended at the bottom. If you cannot pull yourself up from a fully extended position or you cannot pull yourself high enough, you are not strong enough to do this exercise yet. You may need the help of a spotter.

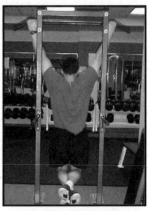

START

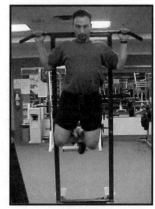

FINISH

DIFFICULTY -	⊢⊣ ⊢⊣	
♂	STARTING WEIGHT - no weight	
♀	STARTING WEIGHT - no weight	

NARROW GRIP PULL-UPS (CHINS)

MAJOR MUSCLES IN USE:
Latissimus Dorsi, Teres Major, Biceps Brachii, Brachialis

STARTING POSITION:
- Standing at the chin-up bar, take an overhand grip so that your hands are positioned directly above your shoulders.
- While hanging with your arms straight, stabilize your shoulders by tensing the shoulder and back muscles.

EXERCISE MOVEMENT:
- As you pull yourself up, raise your chest and lean back slightly to allow the back muscles to do the lifting.
- Try to touch your upper chest to the handle. If this is not possible, you should be able to lift yourself high enough so that your chin is level with the bar.
- Lower yourself back to the starting position so that your arms are straight.

EXERCISE TECHNIQUE POINTS:
- Do not round your back by allowing your chest to lower while pulling up.
- Make sure you pull yourself up smoothly without any jerking or kicking movements.
- Make sure your arms are straight at the beginning of each repetition. If you cannot pull yourself up from a straight arm position or you cannot pull yourself high enough, you are not strong enough to do this exercise yet.

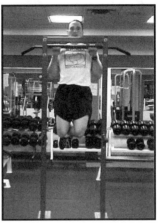

START

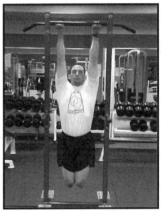

FINISH

DIFFICULTY -	H	H
♂ STARTING WEIGHT - no weight		
♀ STARTING WEIGHT - no weight		

BACK EXERCISES 111

STIFF ARM PULLDOWN

MAJOR MUSCLES IN USE:
Latissimus Dorsi, Teres Major, Trapezius, Serratus Anterior

STARTING POSITION:
- Stand about 2 feet in front of the Pulldown machine with your knees slightly bent, take an overhand grip with hands about shoulder width apart on a long bar.
- Begin with arms slightly bent and your chest up. Lean forward at the waist so that your arms and torso form a straight line.

EXERCISE MOVEMENT:
- While keeping your arms slightly bent and your torso as stationary as possible, pull the bar downwards in a semicircular arc using just your torso strength.
- Pull the bar down until it touches your upper thighs. Reverse the motion so that the bar follows the same path as when it was lowered.

EXERCISE TECHNIQUE POINTS:
- Keep your chest up so that you have a slight arch in your lower back.
- Do not lean too far forward at the end of the motion in order to complete the repetition.
- Make sure your elbows are bent slightly in order to focus the movement more on the back muscles instead of the triceps muscles.
- You may also use the rope handle for this exercise.

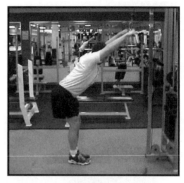

START

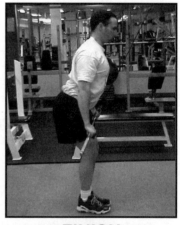

FINISH

DIFFICULTY -	H	H	H
♂ STARTING WEIGHT - 40			
♀ STARTING WEIGHT - 20			

SINGLE STIFF ARM PULLDOWN

MAJOR MUSCLES IN USE:
Latissimus Dorsi, Teres Major, Trapezius, Serratus Anterior

STARTING POSITION:
- Stand about 2 feet in front of the Pulldown machine with your knees slightly bent, take an overhand grip on a single handle.
- Begin with your arm slightly bent and your chest up. Lean forward at the waist so that your arm and torso form a straight line. Place your other hand on your hip.

EXERCISE MOVEMENT:
- While keeping your arm slightly bent and your torso as stationary as possible, pull the handle downwards in a semicircular arc using just your torso strength.
- Pull the handle down until it touches your upper thigh. Reverse the motion so that your arm follows the same path as when it was lowered.

EXERCISE TECHNIQUE POINTS:
- Keep your chest up so that you have a slight arch in your lower back.
- Do not lean too far forward at the end of the motion in order to complete the repetition.
- Make sure your elbow is bent slightly in order to focus the movement more on the back muscles instead of the triceps muscles.
- You may use one side of a rope handle for this exercise

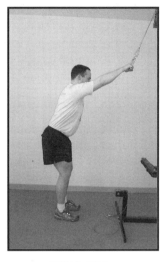

START

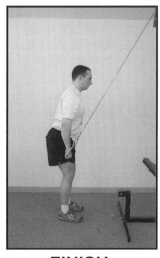

FINISH

DIFFICULTY -	⊢⊣ ⊢⊣ ⊢⊣		
♂	STARTING WEIGHT - 20		
♀	STARTING WEIGHT - 10		

BACK EXERCISES   113

STIFF ARM PULLOVER

MAJOR MUSCLES IN USE:
Latissimus Dorsi, Teres Major, Trapezius

STARTING POSITION:
- Lie on a flat bench. Position a barbell directly over your shoulders using an overhand grip with hands about shoulder width apart. Your arms should have a slight bend at the elbows.

EXERCISE MOVEMENT:
- While keeping your arms slightly bent and your torso as stationary as possible, lower the bar over the top of your head along a semicircular path away from your body using just your torso strength.
- Lower the bar until your upper arms are parallel to the floor. Reverse the motion so that the bar follows the same path as when it was lowered.

EXERCISE TECHNIQUE POINTS:
- Keep your hips on the bench and your torso as stationary as possible.
- Make sure your elbows are bent slightly in order to focus more of the action on the back muscles instead of the triceps muscles.

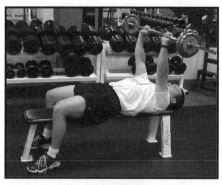
START

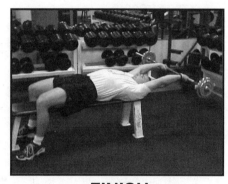
FINISH

DIFFICULTY -	H H H	
♂	STARTING WEIGHT - 25	
♀	STARTING WEIGHT - 15	

DUMBBELL STIFF ARM PULLOVER

MAJOR MUSCLES IN USE:
Latissimus Dorsi, Teres Major, Trapezius

STARTING POSITION:
* Lie on a flat bench. With a dumbbell in each hand, position them directly above your shoulders using an overhand grip with hands about shoulder width apart. Your arms should have a slight bend at the elbows.

EXERCISE MOVEMENT:
* While keeping your arms slightly bent and your torso as stationary as possible, lower the dumbbells over the top of your head along a semicircular path away from your body using just your torso strength.
* Lower the dumbbells until your upper arms are parallel to the floor. Reverse the motion so that the bar follows the same path as when it was lowered.

EXERCISE TECHNIQUE POINTS:
* Keep your hips on the bench and your torso as stationary as possible.
* Make sure your elbows are bent slightly in order to focus more of the action on the back muscles instead of the triceps muscles.
* Do not allow the dumbbells to twist as you raise or lower the weights.
* Try to lower the weight as close to parallel to the floor as you can with each repetition.
* You can also try this exercise with alternate arms or with one arm at a time.

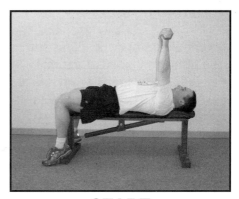

START

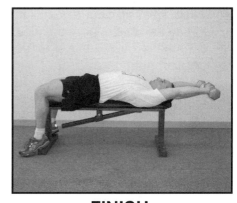

FINISH

DIFFICULTY -	⊢⊣	⊢⊣	⊢⊣
♂ STARTING WEIGHT - 15			
♀ STARTING WEIGHT - 8			

BALL DUMBBELL STIFF ARM PULLOVER

MAJOR MUSCLES IN USE:
Latissimus Dorsi, Teres Major, Trapezius

STARTING POSITION:
- Lie on an exercise ball and position your shoulders and the lower portion of your neck on the highest point of the ball.
- Keep both feet flat on the floor and you hips held high so your shoulders, hips and knees are in a straight line.
- With a dumbbell in each hand, position them directly above your shoulders using an overhand grip with hands about shoulder-width apart. Your arms should have a slight bend at the elbows.

EXERCISE MOVEMENT:
- While keeping your arms slightly bent and your torso as stationary as possible, lower the dumbbells over the top of your head along a circular path away from your body using just your torso strength.
- Lower the dumbbells until your upper arms are parallel to the floor. Reverse the motion so that the bar follows the same path as when it was lowered.

EXERCISE TECHNIQUE POINTS:
- To help keep your torso stable, tense your abdominal and lower back muscles.
- Make sure your elbows are bent slightly in order to focus more of the action on the back muscles instead of the triceps muscles.
- Do not allow the dumbbells to twist as you raise or lower the weights.
- Try to lower the weight as close to parallel to the floor as you can with each repetition.
- You can also perform this exercise with alternating arms or with one arm at a time.

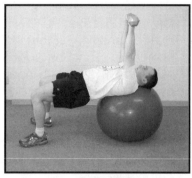
START

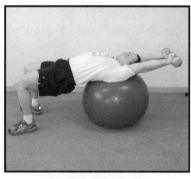
FINISH

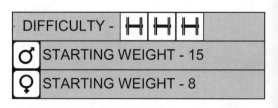

DIFFICULTY -	H	H	H
♂ STARTING WEIGHT - 15			
♀ STARTING WEIGHT - 8			

PRONE DUMBBELL PULLOVER

MAJOR MUSCLES IN USE:
Latissimus Dorsi, Teres Major, Posterior Deltoid, Trapezius, Triceps Brachii

STARTING POSITION:
- Position yourself on a high bench (either a specially designed adjustable bench or a normal bench on blocks) so that you are lying on your stomach with your arms hanging down on either side. Your fingers should not touch the floor.
- In each hand grasp a dumbbell and allow the dumbbells to hang directly below your shoulders with your arms straight and palms facing back towards your feet.

EXERCISE MOVEMENT:
- While keeping your elbows in a slightly bent position, start by moving the dumbbells back along the side of your body in an upwards arc by only allowing movement at your shoulder joint.
- Your arm should swing alongside your body like a pendulum while your hand twists upwards.
- At the end point in the movement your hand should be level with your hip and your palm facing upwards.
- Finish the exercise by returning the dumbbell to the starting position along the same path that it was raised.

EXERCISE TECHNIQUE POINTS:
- Keep your hips on the bench and your torso as stationary as possible.
- Make sure your elbows are bent slightly in order to focus more of the action on the back muscles instead of the triceps muscles.
- You may also start this movement with your palms facing each other.

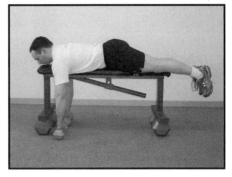

START

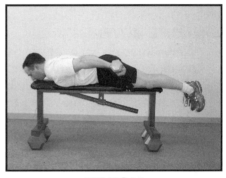

FINISH

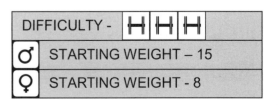

DIFFICULTY -	⊢⊢ ⊢⊢ ⊢⊢	
♂	STARTING WEIGHT – 15	
♀	STARTING WEIGHT - 8	

DUMBBELL BENT OVER PULLOVER

MAJOR MUSCLES IN USE:
Latissimus Dorsi, Teres Major, Posterior Deltoid, Trapezius, Triceps Brachii

STARTING POSITION:
- Stand with your feet about shoulder width apart and your knees slightly bent.
- Bend over at the waist with your hips and buttocks pushed out forming a slight curve in your lower back. Your upper back should be flat. Your upper back will flatten if you keep your chest up.
- Grasp two dumbbells and position your hands so that your palms are facing back towards your feet. Your abdominal muscles should be tensed. Your upper back should be just above parallel to the floor.

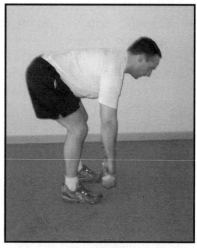

START

EXERCISE MOVEMENT:
- While keeping your elbows in a slightly bent position, start by moving the dumbbells back along the side of your body in an upwards arc by only allowing movement at your shoulder joint.
- Your arm should swing alongside your body like a pendulum while your hand twists upwards.
- At the end point in the movement your hand should be level with your hip and your palm facing upwards.
- Finish the exercise by returning the dumbbell to the starting position along the same path that it was raised.

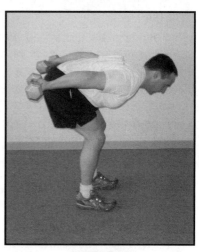

FINISH

EXERCISE TECHNIQUE POINTS:
- Keep your hips on the bench and your torso as stationary as possible.
- Make sure your elbows are bent slightly in order to focus more of the action on the back muscles instead of the triceps muscles.
- You may also start this movement with your palms facing each other.
- You can also try this exercise with alternating arms or one arm at a time.

DIFFICULTY -	H H H	
♂	STARTING WEIGHT – 15	
♀	STARTING WEIGHT - 8	

CABLE STIFF ARM PULLOVER

MAJOR MUSCLES IN USE:

Latissimus Dorsi, Teres Major, Triceps Brachii, Pectoralis Major, Serratus Anterior

STARTING POSITION:

- Lie flat on your back on an exercise bench and hold a bar attached to a low pulley directly above your chest with your arms just slightly bent at the elbows. Your hands should be spaced about shoulder-width apart.

EXERCISE MOVEMENT:

- While keeping your elbows locked in a slightly bent position, lower the bar as shown in the pictures on the right side of the page. The bar should travel over your head and away from your body.
- Lower the bar down as far as possible and then lift it back to the starting position along the same path than when it was lowered.

EXERCISE TECHNIQUE POINTS:

- Keep your body as still as possible and try not to arch your lower back too much or let your feet come off the ground.
- Try to keep your elbows in the same position as when you started.
- Make sure your elbows are slightly bent in order to focus the movement more on the upper body muscles.

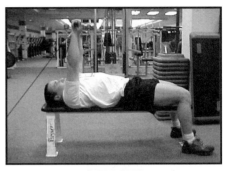

START

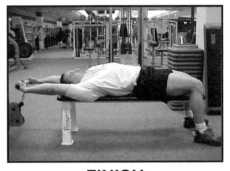

FINISH

DIFFICULTY -	⊢⊣	⊢⊣	⊢⊣
♂	STARTING WEIGHT - 40		
♀	STARTING WEIGHT - 20		

BENT OVER ROW

MAJOR MUSCLES IN USE:
Latissimus Dorsi, Teres Major, Biceps Brachii, Brachialis, Erector Spinae

STARTING POSITION:
- Stand with feet wider than shoulder width apart and your knees slightly bent.
- Bend over at the waist with your hips and buttocks pushed out, forming a slight curve in your lower back. Your upper back should be flat. Your upper back will flatten if you keep your chest up.
- Grasp the bar with a shoulder-width, overhand grip. Keep the bar close to your legs. Your abdominal muscles should be tensed. Your upper back should be just above parallel to the floor.

EXERCISE MOVEMENT:
- While keeping your upper back stationary and your abdominal muscles tensed, lift the bar up by pulling it towards your navel.
- Raise the bar until it lightly touches your midsection. Reverse the motion so that the bar follows the same path back to the starting position.

EXERCISE TECHNIQUE POINTS:
- Keep your chest and buttocks pushed out so that you have a slight arch in your lower back while your upper back remains flat.
- Do not allow your upper body to rise as if you were beginning to stand up.
- Make sure you pull the bar up towards your navel.
- You may wish to wear a belt on this exercise to help support the trunk.

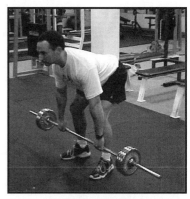

START

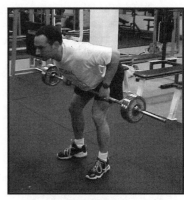

FINISH

DIFFICULTY -	H H H H
♂ STARTING WEIGHT - 65	
♀ STARTING WEIGHT - 35	

BACK EXERCISES

CABLE BENT OVER ROW

MAJOR MUSCLES IN USE:

Latissimus Dorsi, Teres Major, Biceps Brachii, Brachialis, Erector Spinae

STARTING POSITION:

- Stand with feet wider than shoulder width apart and your knees slightly bent in front of a long bar attached to the low pulley of a pulley machine.
- Bend over at the waist with your hips and buttocks pushed out, forming a slight curve in your lower back. Your upper back should be flat. Your upper back will flatten if you keep your chest up.
- Grasp the bar with a shoulder-width, overhand grip. Your abdominal muscles should be tensed. Your upper back should be just above parallel to the floor. You should be leaning back onto your heels slightly to compensate for the weight.

EXERCISE MOVEMENT:

- While keeping your upper back stationary and your abdominal muscles tensed, pull the bar up and towards your navel.
- Raise the bar until it lightly touches your midsection. Reverse the motion so that the bar follows the same path back to the starting position.

EXERCISE TECHNIQUE POINTS:

- Keep your chest and buttocks pushed out so that you have a slight arch in your lower back while your upper back remains flat.
- Do not allow your upper body to rise as if you were beginning to stand up.
- Make sure you pull the bar up towards your navel.
- You may wish to wear a belt on this exercise to help support the trunk.
- To help counteract the feeling of being pulled forward as you do the exercise, lean back onto you heels by pushing your hips further back.

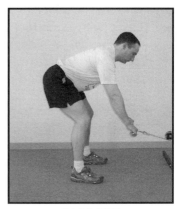

START

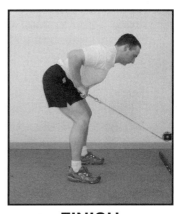

FINISH

DIFFICULTY -	H	H	H	H
♂ STARTING WEIGHT - 65				
♀ STARTING WEIGHT - 35				

REVERSE GRIP BENT OVER ROW

MAJOR MUSCLES IN USE:

Latissimus Dorsi, Teres Major, Biceps Brachii, Brachialis, Erector Spinae

STARTING POSITION:

- Stand with your feet slightly wider apart than shoulder width and your knees slightly bent. Bend over at the waist so that your hips and buttocks are pushed out allowing a slight curve in the lower back. Your upper back should be flat. Your upper back will flatten if you keep your chest pushed out.
- Grasp the bar with a wider than shoulder-width underhand grip, allowing it to hang close to your legs. Your abdominal muscles should be tensed. Your upper body should be at about a 25° angle to the floor.

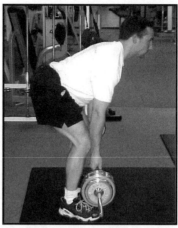

START

EXERCISE MOVEMENT:

- While keeping your upper back stationary and your abdominal muscles tensed, pull the bar up towards your navel. Make sure you try to keep your elbows tucked in at your sides as you lift the barbell.
- Pull the bar up until it lightly touches your midsection. Reverse the motion so that the bar follows the same path as it was lifted.

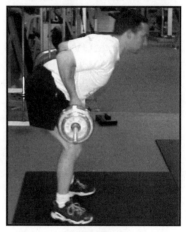

FINISH

EXERCISE TECHNIQUE POINTS:

- Keep your chest and buttocks pushed out so that you have a slight arch in your lower back and your upper back remains flat.
- Do not allow your upper body to rise as if you were going to stand up. A slight sway in the torso is acceptable.
- Make sure you pull the bar up towards your navel and not towards the chest.
- You may wish to wear a belt on this exercise to help support the trunk.

DIFFICULTY -	H H H H
♂ STARTING WEIGHT - 65	
♀ STARTING WEIGHT - 35	

DUMBBELL BENT OVER ROW

MAJOR MUSCLES IN USE:
Latissimus Dorsi, Teres Major, Biceps Brachii, Brachialis, Erector Spinae

STARTING POSITION:
- Stand with feet about shoulde -width apart and your knees slightly bent.
- Bend over at the waist with your hips and buttocks pushed out forming a slight curve in your lower back. Your upper back should be flat. Your upper back will flatten if you keep your chest up.
- Grasp two dumbbells and position your hands so that your palms are facing each other while your arms are straight. Your abdominal muscles should be tensed. Your upper back should be just above parallel to the floor.

EXERCISE MOVEMENT:
- While keeping your upper body stationary and your back flat, pull the dumbbells up towards the sides of your hips. Make sure you try and keep your elbows tucked in close to your sides.
- Pull the dumbbells up until the rear bell of the dumbbell lightly touches your hip. Reverse the motion by lowering the dumbbell down and forward so that the dumbbells return to the starting position.

EXERCISE TECHNIQUE POINTS:
- Keep your chest and buttocks pushed out so that you have a slight arch in your lower back while your upper back remains flat.
- Do not allow your upper body to rise as if you were beginning to stand up.
- You may wish to wear a belt on this exercise to help support the trunk.

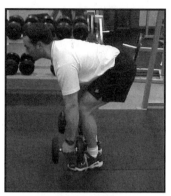

START

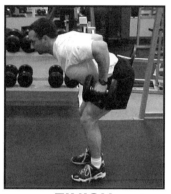

FINISH

DIFFICULTY -	H H H		
♂	STARTING WEIGHT - 25		
♀	STARTING WEIGHT - 15		

SEATED ROW (CLOSE GRIP)

MAJOR MUSCLES IN USE:
Latissimus Dorsi, Teres Major, Biceps Brachii, Brachialis, Erector Spinae

STARTING POSITION:
- Sit in front of a low pulley with your feet placed on either side and about 6 inches in front of the pulley. Many commercial gyms have a specialized machine to do this specific movement.
- Grasp the Close Grip handle and sit up straight with your chest high and your knees slightly bent. Your torso should stay in this position throughout the exercise set.

EXERCISE MOVEMENT:
- While keeping your torso stationary and your abdominal muscles tensed, pull the handle towards your belt line. Make sure you try and keep your elbows tucked in close to your sides.
- Pull the handle in until it lightly touches your midsection. Reverse the motion so that the handle returns to the same position as when you began.

EXERCISE TECHNIQUE POINTS:
- Straighten your back and keep your chest high so that you have a slight arch in your lower back.
- Do not allow yourself to sway excessively when performing your repetitions. A very slight swaying of the torso is acceptable; too much swaying may indicate you are using a weight that is too heavy.
- Make sure you pull the handle towards your belt line and not towards the chest.

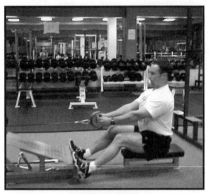

START

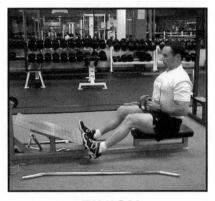

FINISH

DIFFICULTY -	⊢⊣ ⊢⊣	
♂	STARTING WEIGHT - 70	
♀	STARTING WEIGHT - 40	

BACK EXERCISES

SEATED BAR ROW (WIDE GRIP)

MAJOR MUSCLES IN USE:
Latissimus Dorsi, Teres Major, Biceps Brachii, Brachialis Erector Spinae,

STARTING POSITION:
- Sitting in front of a low pulley, place your feet on either side of the cable about 6 inches in front of the pulley. Many commercial gyms a specialized machine to do this specific movement.
- Grasp a long bar handle with your hands placed a little wider apart than shoulder-width. Sit up straight with your chest high and your knees bent. Your torso should stay in this position throughout the exercise.

EXERCISE MOVEMENT:
- While keeping your torso stationary and your abdominal muscles tensed, pull the bar towards the middle of your abdominal region. Allow your elbows to follow their natural movement path backwards.
- Pull the handle in until it lightly touches your midsection. Reverse the motion so that the handle returns to the same place as when you began your repetition.

EXERCISE TECHNIQUE POINTS:
- Straighten your back by keeping your chest high so that you have a slight arch in your lower back.
- Do not allow yourself to sway excessively when performing your repetitions. A very slight swaying of the torso is acceptable. However, too much may indicate you are using a weight that is too heavy.
- Make sure you pull the bar towards the middle of your abdominal region.
- Do not allow your wrists to bend near the end of the motion.

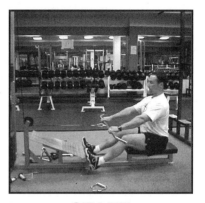

START

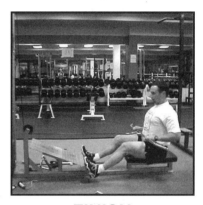

FINISH

DIFFICULTY -	H	H	
♂	STARTING WEIGHT - 70		
♀	STARTING WEIGHT - 40		

BACK EXERCISES 125

SEATED ROPE ROW

MAJOR MUSCLES IN USE:
Latissimus Dorsi, Teres Major, Biceps Brachii, Brachialis, Erector Spinae

STARTING POSITION:
*   Sit in front of a low pulley with your feet placed on either side and about 6 inches in front of the pulley. Many commercial gyms have a specialized machine to do this specific movement.
*   Grasp the rope handles on each end and sit up straight with your chest high and your knees slightly bent. Your torso should stay in this position throughout the exercise.

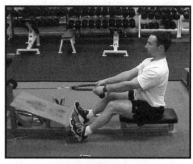

START

EXERCISE MOVEMENT:
*   While keeping your torso stationary and your abdominal muscles tensed, pull the handles towards your belt line so that your hands go to either side of your torso. Make sure you try and keep your elbows tucked in close to your sides.
*   Pull the handles in until they lightly touch both sides of your midsection. Reverse the motion so that the handles return to the same position as when you began.

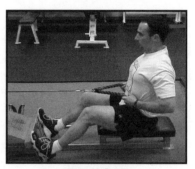

FINISH

EXERCISE TECHNIQUE POINTS:
*   Straighten your back and keep your chest high so that you have a slight arch in your lower back.
*   Do not allow yourself to sway excessively when performing your repetitions. A very slight swaying of the torso is acceptable. However, too much swaying may indicate that you are using a weight that is too heavy.
*   Make sure you pull the handle towards your belt line and not towards the chest.

DIFFICULTY -	⊢⊣ ⊢⊣ ⊢⊣	
♂	STARTING WEIGHT - 70	
♀	STARTING WEIGHT - 40	

BACK EXERCISES

ONE ARM CABLE ROW

MAJOR MUSCLES IN USE:
Latissimus Dorsi, Teres Major, Biceps Brachii, Brachialis Erector Spinae,

STARTING POSITION:
- Sit in front of a low pulley with your feet placed on either side and about 6 inches in front of the pulley. Many commercial gyms a specialized machine to do this specific movement.
- Using one hand, grasp a single handle and sit up straight with your chest high and your knees slightly bent. Your torso should stay in this position throughout the whole set.

EXERCISE MOVEMENT:
- While keeping your torso stationary and your abdominal muscles tensed, pull the handle towards your side at the level of the belt line. Make sure you try and keep your elbow tucked in close to your side.
- Pull the handle in until it lightly touches your midsection. Reverse the motion so that the handle returns to the same place as when you began your repetition.

EXERCISE TECHNIQUE POINTS:
- Straighten your back by keeping your chest high so that you have a slight arch in your lower back.
- Do not allow yourself to sway or twist excessively when performing your repetitions. A slight sway or twist of the torso is acceptable; however, too much may indicate you are using a weight that is too heavy.
- Make sure you pull the handle towards your belt line and not towards the chest.

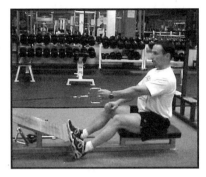

START

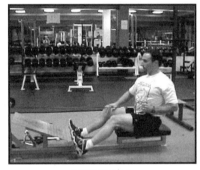

FINISH

DIFFICULTY -	H	H	H
♂ STARTING WEIGHT - 40			
♀ STARTING WEIGHT - 20			

STANDING ONE ARM CABLE ROW

MAJOR MUSCLES IN USE:
Latissimus Dorsi, Teres Major, Biceps Brachii, Brachialis, Erector Spinae

STARTING POSITION:
- Stand several feet in front of a low pulley and place one foot in front of the other. With one hand, grasp a single handle and lean forward slightly with your chest high and your knees slightly bent. Your torso should stay in this position throughout the whole set. Place your other hand on your hip or thigh.

EXERCISE MOVEMENT:
- While keeping your torso stationary and your abdominal muscles tensed, pull the handle towards your side to the level of the belt line. Make sure you try and keep your elbow tucked in close to your side.
- Pull the handle in until it lightly touches your midsection. Reverse the motion so that the handle returns to the same place as when you began your repetition.

EXERCISE TECHNIQUE POINTS:
- Straighten your back by keeping your chest high so that you have a slight arch in your lower back.
- Do not allow yourself to sway or twist excessively when performing your repetitions. A slight sway or twist of the torso is acceptable, however too much may indicate you are using a weight that is too heavy.
- Make sure you pull the handle towards your belt line and not towards the chest.

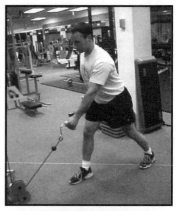

START

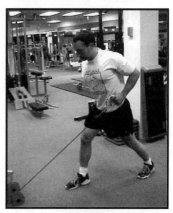

FINISH

DIFFICULTY -	H	H	H
♂	STARTING WEIGHT - 40		
♀	STARTING WEIGHT - 20		

ONE ARM ROW

MAJOR MUSCLES IN USE:
Latissimus Dorsi, Teres Major, Biceps Brachii, Brachialis, Erector Spinae

STARTING POSITION:
- Support yourself on a bench by placing the same knee and hand on one side of a flat bench. The other foot should be placed on the floor while the other hand holds the dumbbell.
- Allow the dumbbell to hang directly below your shoulder with your arm straight. Your back should be flat and shoulders level with the floor.

EXERCISE MOVEMENT:
- While keeping your upper body stationary and your back flat, pull the dumbbell up towards the side of your hip. Make sure you try and keep your elbow tucked in close to your side.
- Pull the dumbbell up until the rear bell of the dumbbell lightly touches your hip. Reverse the motion by lowering the dumbbell down and forward so that the dumbbell returns to the same place as when you began.

EXERCISE TECHNIQUE POINTS:
- Keep your upper back flat with a slight arch in your lower back.
- Do not allow your torso to sway or twist excessively when performing the repetitions. Be careful not to twist the shoulders excessively as this can put unnecessary strain on your back muscles.
- Make sure you pull the handle towards your hip and belt line and not towards the chest.

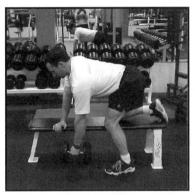

START

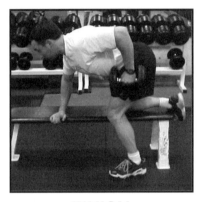

FINISH

DIFFICULTY -	⊢⊣ ⊢⊣ ⊢
♂ STARTING WEIGHT - 25	
♀ STARTING WEIGHT - 12	

T-BAR ROW

MAJOR MUSCLES IN USE:
Latissimus Dorsi, Teres Major, Biceps Brachii, Brachialis, Erector Spinae

STARTING POSITION:
- Straddle the end of a long barbell with your feet placed slightly wider apart than shoulder width. You should be facing the weight plates that are loaded on only one end of the bar. Use a short bar with a slight bend or groove in the middle (a standard triceps bar handle works well). The long bar should be placed in the groove at the bottom of the "V" of the handle.
- Bend your knees and bend over at the waist so that your hips and buttocks are pushed out allowing a slight curve in the lower back. Your upper back should be straight and at about 30° - 40° to the floor.
- Grasp the bar with an overhand grip and lift the end of the bar up off the floor using your legs. Your knees should remain slightly bent.

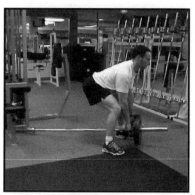

START

EXERCISE MOVEMENT:
- While keeping your upper back stationary and your abdominal muscles tensed, pull the bar up towards your midsection. The opposite end of the bar is to remain in contact with the floor.
- Lower the bar along the same path that it was lifted.

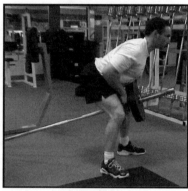

FINISH

EXERCISE TECHNIQUE POINTS:
- Keep your chest and buttocks pushed out so that you have a slight arch in your lower back and your upper back remains flat.
- Do not allow yourself to raise your upper body upwards.
- If the other end of the bar rises off the ground, try to sit back a little more or place a moderately heavy dumbbell across the end.
- You may wish to wear a belt for this exercise to help support the lower back.

DIFFICULTY -	⊢ ⊢ ⊢ ⊦
♂ STARTING WEIGHT - 60	
♀ STARTING WEIGHT - 30	

DUMBELL BENCH ROW

MAJOR MUSCLES IN USE:
Latissimus Dorsi, Teres Major, Biceps Brachii, Brachialis, Erector Spinae

STARTING POSITION:
- Position yourself on a high bench (either a specially designed adjustable bench or a normal bench on blocks) so that you are lying on your stomach with your arms hanging down on either side. Your fingers should not touch the floor.
- In each hand grasp a dumbbell and allow the dumbbells to hang directly below your shoulders when your arms are straight.

EXERCISE MOVEMENT:
- While keeping your elbows and upper arms tucked in, pull the dumbbells up with both arms towards the sides of your torso.
- The dumbbells should rise towards your belt line until they lightly touch the bench. Reverse the motion by lowering the dumbbell down and forward so that your hand returns to the same place as when you began.

EXERCISE TECHNIQUE POINTS:
- Do not round your upper back. Make sure it stays parallel with the bench while maintaining a slight arch in your lower back.
- Do not allow yourself to twist or arch your upper body so that your chest rises off the bench when performing your repetitions.
- Make sure you pull the handle of the dumbbell towards your belt line and not towards the chest.

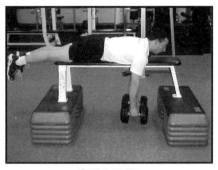

START

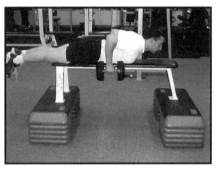

FINISH

DIFFICULTY -	H	H	H
♂ STARTING WEIGHT - 25			
♀ STARTING WEIGHT - 12			

BACK EXERCISES

TRAPEZIUS EXERCISES

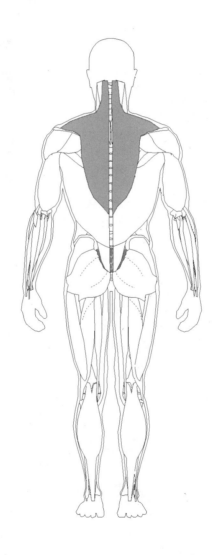

BARBELL SHRUGS

MAJOR MUSCLES IN USE:
Trapezius

STARTING POSITION:
- Take an overhand, shoulder-width grip on a barbell.
- Shoulders are held back and your chest is held high.
- Tense the abdominal and lower back muscles.

EXERCISE MOVEMENT:
- Begin the movement by raising your shoulders directly upwards as high as possible while keeping your arms straight.
- When you cannot raise your shoulders any higher, lower the weight back down so that the bar is once again resting against your upper thighs.

EXERCISE TECHNIQUE POINTS:
- Straighten your back by keeping your chest up and shoulders back.
- Do not bounce in the bottom position.
- Do not allow your legs to bend in order to help you lift the weight.
- Do not roll your shoulders forwards or backwards as you perform the movement.
- Make sure that you lift the weight as high as you can. This will help ensure that you are getting the fullest range possible.

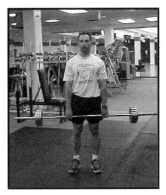

START

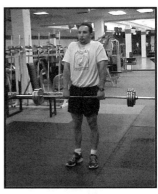

FINISH

DIFFICULTY -	H	
♂	STARTING WEIGHT - 85	
♀	STARTING WEIGHT - 55	

TRAPEZIUS EXERCISES 133

BEHIND-THE-BACK BARBELL SHRUGS

MAJOR MUSCLES IN USE:
Trapezius

STARTING POSITION:
- Hold a barbell against the backs of your thighs by taking an underhand grip about shoulder width apart. Your palms should be facing away from your body.
- Shoulders are held back and your chest is held high.
- Tense the abdominal and lower back muscles.

EXERCISE MOVEMENT:
- Begin the movement by raising your shoulders directly upwards as high as possible while keeping your arms straight.
- When you can no longer raise your shoulders any higher, lower the weight back to the starting position.

EXERCISE TECHNIQUE POINTS:
- Straighten your back by keeping your chest up and shoulders back.
- Do not bounce in the bottom position.
- Do not allow your legs to bend in order to help you lift the weight.
- Do not roll your shoulders forwards or backwards as you perform the movement.
- Make sure that you lift the weight as high as you can. This will help ensure that you are getting the fullest range possible.

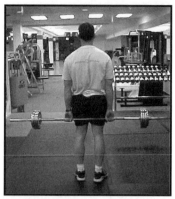

START

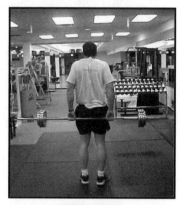

FINISH

DIFFICULTY -	H	H
♂ STARTING WEIGHT - 85		
♀ STARTING WEIGHT - 55		

TRAPEZIUS EXERCISES

DUMBBELL SHRUGS

MAJOR MUSCLES IN USE:

Trapezius

STARTING POSITION:

- Stand holding a dumbbell in each hand with your palms facing the sides of your thighs.
- Shoulders are held back and your chest is held high.
- Tense the abdominal and lower back muscles.

EXERCISE MOVEMENT:

- Begin the movement by raising your shoulders directly upwards as high as possible while keeping your arms straight.
- When you can no longer raise your shoulders higher, lower the weight back to the starting position.

EXERCISE TECHNIQUE POINTS:

- Straighten your back by keeping your chest up and shoulders back.
- Do not bounce in the bottom position.
- Do not allow your legs to bend in order to help you lift the weight.
- Do not roll your shoulders forwards or backwards as you perform the movement.
- Make sure that you lift the weight as high as you can. This will help ensure that you are getting the fullest range possible.

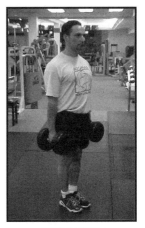

START

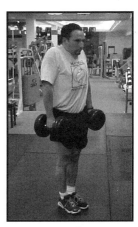

FINISH

DIFFICULTY - ⊢⊣	
♂	STARTING WEIGHT - 40
♀	STARTING WEIGHT - 20

TRAPEZIUS EXERCISES

SEATED DUMBBELL SHRUGS

MAJOR MUSCLES IN USE:
 Trapezius

STARTING POSITION:
- While holding a dumbbell in each hand, sit at the end of a bench. Your hands should hang below the level of the bench seat and your palms should face each other.
- Shoulders are held back and your chest is held high.

EXERCISE MOVEMENT:
- Begin the movement by raising your shoulders directly upwards as high as possible while keeping your arms straight.
- When you can no longer raise your shoulders any higher, lower the weight back to the starting position.

EXERCISE TECHNIQUE POINTS:
- Straighten your back by keeping your chest up and shoulders back.
- Do not bounce in the bottom position.
- Do not roll your shoulders forwards or backwards as you perform the movement.
- Make sure that you lift the weight as high as you can. This will help ensure that you are getting the fullest range possible.

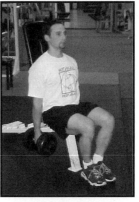

START

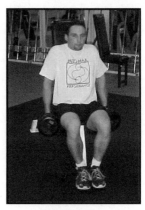

FINISH

DIFFICULTY -	H	
♂	STARTING WEIGHT - 35	
♀	STARTING WEIGHT - 20	

ONE ARM CABLE SHRUGS

MAJOR MUSCLES IN USE:
Trapezius

STARTING POSITION:
- Stand holding a single handle attached to the low pulley of a pulley machine. Your palm should be facing in towards your thighs.
- Place your unused hand on your hip or flat against your upper thigh.
- Shoulders are held back with your chest up.
- Tense the abdominal and lower back muscles.

EXERCISE MOVEMENT:
- Begin the movement by lifting your shoulder (of the arm holding the handle) directly upwards as high as possible while keeping your arm straight.
- When you can no longer raise your shoulder any higher, lower the weight back to the starting position.

EXERCISE TECHNIQUE POINTS:
- Straighten your back by keeping your chest up and shoulders back.
- Do not bounce in the bottom position.
- Do not allow your legs to bend in order to help you lift the weight.
- Do not roll your shoulders forwards or backwards as you perform the movement.
- Make sure that you lift the weight as high as you can. This will help ensure that you are getting the fullest range possible.
- Do not lean to one side in order to complete the necessary repetitions.

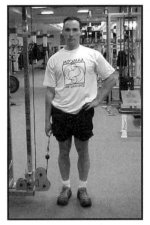

START

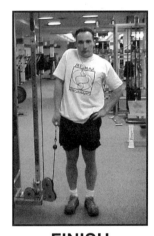

FINISH

DIFFICULTY -	⊢⊣	⊢⊣
♂ STARTING WEIGHT - 45		
♀ STARTING WEIGHT - 20		

CABLE REAR SHRUGS

MAJOR MUSCLES IN USE:
Trapezius

STARTING POSITION:
- Sit at a low pulley or at a seated row machine and take an overhand grip on the close grip handle with your palms facing each other.
- Begin with arms held straight, keeping your chest up and your torso at a 90° angle to the floor.

EXERCISE MOVEMENT:
- While holding your arms straight in front of you, pull your shoulders back and squeeze your shoulder blades together.
- Return the handle to the starting position. At the end of the movement your shoulders should be slightly rounded and pulled forward. Repeat the movement again for the desired number of repetitions.

EXERCISE TECHNIQUE POINTS:
- Do not swing or rock back and forth in order to complete the repetitions.
- Always make sure your elbows are completely straight.
- Round the shoulders but do not round the back.

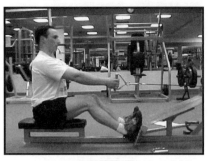

START

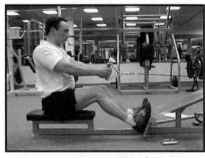

FINISH

DIFFICULTY -	⊢ ⊢ ⊢	
♂	STARTING WEIGHT - 60	
♀	STARTING WEIGHT - 30	

TRAPEZIUS EXERCISES

ONE ARM CABLE REAR SHRUGS

MAJOR MUSCLES IN USE:
Trapezius

STARTING POSITION:
- Standing or sitting at a pulldown machine, take an overhand grip on a single handle with your palm facing inwards.
- Begin with the arm straight, elbow locked, and chest up. Lean back at a 45° angle if you are sitting. If standing lean back slightly so that the angle between your arm and your torso should form about a 90° - 110° angle.
- Place your other hand on your hip or thigh to help stabilize your upper body.

EXERCISE MOVEMENT:
- While keeping your arm straight, pull your shoulder back and squeeze your shoulder blades together.
- Return the handle back to the starting position so that at the end of the movement your shoulders are slightly rounded and pulled forward. Repeat the movement again for the desired number of repetitions.

EXERCISE TECHNIQUE POINTS:
- Do not swing or rock back and forth in order to complete the repetitions.
- Always make sure your arm is completely straight.
- Round the shoulders but do not round the back.

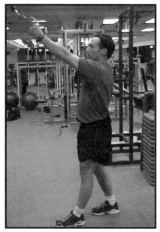

START

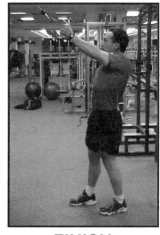

FINISH

DIFFICULTY -	H H H H
♂ STARTING WEIGHT - 30	
♀ STARTING WEIGHT - 15	

LOWER BACK EXERCISES

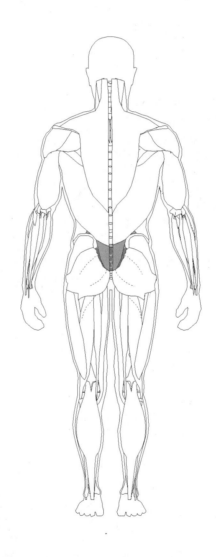

GOOD MORNINGS

MAJOR MUSCLES IN USE:

Erector Spinae, Biceps Femoris, Semitendinosus, Gluteus Maximus

STARTING POSITION:
- Position a barbell across the back of your shoulders.
- Feet should be shoulder-width apart.
- Knees should be slightly bent.
- Shoulders are held back and your chest held high.
- Tense the abdominal and lower back muscles.

EXERCISE MOVEMENT:
- Begin by slowly bending forward, allowing your hips to lead the movement by moving them backwards first.
- End this lowering portion when your back is almost parallel to the floor. At this point reverse the movement until you are once again standing straight.

EXERCISE TECHNIQUE POINTS:
- Your back should always be straight. You can achieve this by keeping your chest up, your shoulders back, and by pushing your buttocks out throughout the whole motion.
- Do not bounce in the bottom position.
- It is normal for your legs to bend slightly in the lowering portion.
- Make sure you keep your back straight by sticking the buttocks out throughout the whole motion.

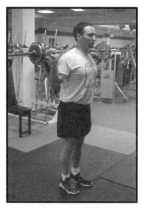

START

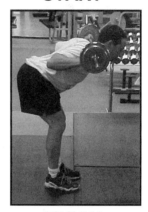

FINISH

DIFFICULTY -	H H H	
♂	STARTING WEIGHT - 35	
♀	STARTING WEIGHT - 15	

LOWER BACK EXERCISES 141

STANDING BACK EXTENSION

MAJOR MUSCLES IN USE:
  Erector Spinae, Biceps Femoris, Semitendinosus, Gluteus Maximus

STARTING POSITION:
- Position a dumbbell across the top of your chest at the base of your neck.
- Feet should be shoulder-width apart.
- Knees should be slightly bent.
- Shoulders are held back and your chest held high.
- Tense the abdominal and lower back muscles.

EXERCISE MOVEMENT:
- Begin by slowly bending forward, allowing your hips to lead the movement by moving them backwards first.
- End this lowering portion when your back is almost parallel to the floor. At this point reverse the movement until you are once again standing straight.

EXERCISE TECHNIQUE POINTS:
- Your back should always be straight. You can achieve this by keeping your chest up, your shoulders back, and by pushing your buttocks out throughout the whole motion.
- Do not bounce in the bottom position.
- It is normal for your legs to bend slightly in the lowering portion.
- Make sure you keep your back straight by sticking the buttocks out throughout the whole motion

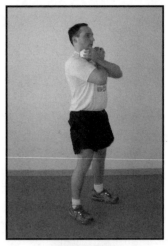

START

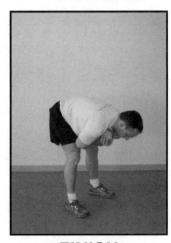

FINISH

DIFFICULTY -	H H H	
♂	STARTING WEIGHT - 25	
♀	STARTING WEIGHT - 12	

LOWER BACK EXERCISES 142

HYPER-EXTENSIONS

MAJOR MUSCLES IN USE:
Erector Spinae, Biceps Femoris, Semitendinosus, Gluteus Maximus

STARTING POSITION:
- Position your hips on the large pad of the hyperextension bench and the backs of your ankles under the small pads. Your ankles should be slightly below the level of your hips.
- Cross your hands over your chest or behind your head and lock your knees.
- Your torso should be hanging down towards the floor.
- Tense the abdominal and lower back muscles.

EXERCISE MOVEMENT:
- Begin the movement by slowly raising your upper body. Lead the movement with your chest and shoulders.
- Finish the exercise movement with your back slightly arched upwards and your torso slightly above a line parallel to the floor.
- Reverse the movement, lowering your upper body back down along the same path to the starting position.

EXERCISE TECHNIQUE POINTS:
- Make sure your back is always straight by keeping your chest up and your shoulders back.
- Do not bounce in the bottom position.
- Do not allow your legs to bend at any point in the motion.
- Make sure you keep your back straight by tensing your abdominal, lower back, hamstring, and buttock muscles.
- You may wish to add a weight behind your head if you find the movement to easy.

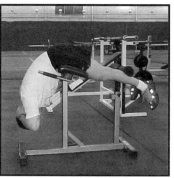

START

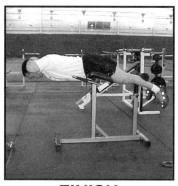

FINISH

DIFFICULTY -	H	H
♂ STARTING WEIGHT – no weight		
♀ STARTING WEIGHT - no weight		

LOWER BACK EXERCISES 143

BALL HYPER-EXTENSIONS

MAJOR MUSCLES IN USE:
Erector Spinae, Biceps Femoris, Semitendinosus, Gluteus Maximus

STARTING POSITION:
- Position your hips on the top portion of an exercise ball and brace your feet against a wall or other sturdy object.
- Cross your hands over your chest or behind your head. You may bend your knees to help in balancing on the ball.
- Your torso should be hanging down towards the floor.
- Tense the abdominal and lower back muscles.

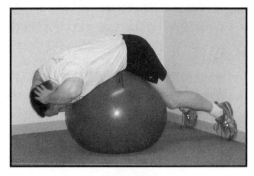

START

EXERCISE MOVEMENT:
- Begin the movement by slowly raising your upper body. Lead the movement with your chest and shoulders.
- Finish the exercise movement with your back slightly arched upwards and your torso slightly above a line parallel to the floor.
- Reverse the movement, lowering your upper body back down along the same path to the starting position.

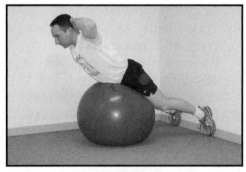

FINISH

EXERCISE TECHNIQUE POINTS:
- Make sure your back is always straight by keeping your chest up and your shoulders back.
- Do not bounce in the bottom position.
- Make sure you keep your back straight by tensing your abdominal, lower back, hamstring, and buttock muscles.
- You may wish to add a weight behind your head if you find the movement to easy.

DIFFICULTY -	H H H I-
♂ STARTING WEIGHT - no weight	
♀ STARTING WEIGHT - no weight	

SEATED BACK EXTENSION

MAJOR MUSCLES IN USE:
Erector Spinae

STARTING POSITION:
- Sit in front of a low pulley with your feet placed on either side and about 6 inches in front of the pulley. Many commercial gyms have a specialised machine to do this specific movement. Grasp a short bar handle and allow your arms to straighten all the way.
- Bend forward while keeping your chest high and your knees slightly bent.

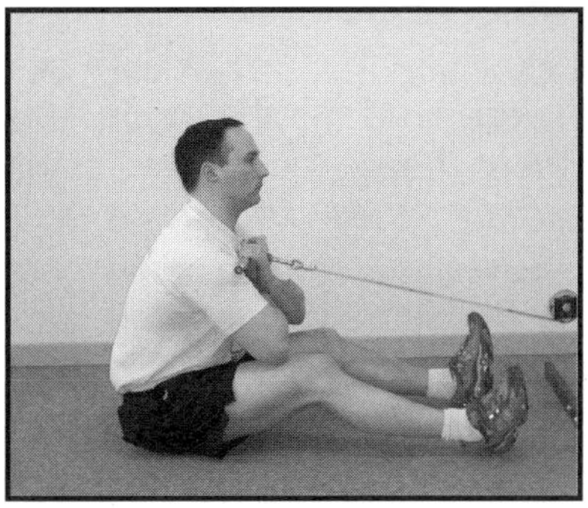

START

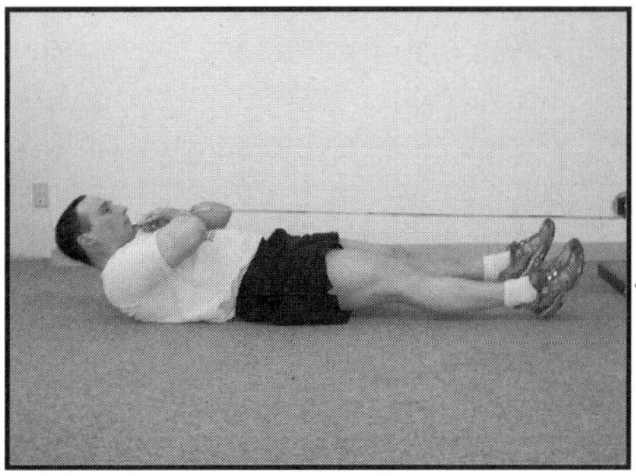

FINISH

EXERCISE MOVEMENT:
- While keeping your chest high and your abdominal muscles tensed, lean backwards using your lower back muscles to pull you back.
- Lean backwards until you are almost lying flat on the bench.
- Reverse the movement, bringing your upper body back along the same path to the starting position.

EXERCISE TECHNIQUE POINTS:
- Straighten your back and keep your chest high throughout the movement.
- Do not allow your knees to straighten as this will put excessive pressure on the discs in your lower back.
- Make sure you keep the handle close to your chest throughout the whole movement. You may wish to experiment with various grips to make it more comfortable.

DIFFICULTY -	2
♂	STARTING WEIGHT - 40
♀	STARTING WEIGHT - 70

STRAIGHT LEG EXTENSIONS

MAJOR MUSCLES IN USE:

Erector Spinae, Biceps Femoris, Semitendinosus, Gluteus Maximus

STARTING POSITION:
- Position the midsection of your torso on the large pad of the hyperextension bench with your head facing the small pads. Your legs should point outwards away from the machine.
- Steady your upper body by grasping the smaller pads or the frame of the machine.
- Your legs should be hanging down towards the floor so that your body is almost at a 90° angle to the floor.
- Tense the abdominal and lower back muscles.

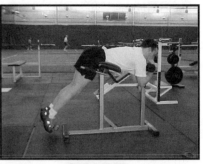

START

EXERCISE MOVEMENT:
- Begin the movement by slowly raising your legs upwards while keeping your knees locked.
- Finish the exercise movement with your legs slightly arched upwards and slightly above a parallel line to the floor.
- Lower your legs back to the starting position along the same path that they were raised.

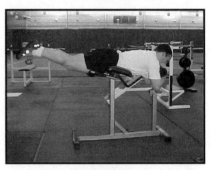

FINISH

EXERCISE TECHNIQUE POINTS:
- Make sure your back is always straight by keeping your chest up and your shoulders back.
- Do not allow your legs to bend at any point in the motion.
- Make sure you keep your back straight by tensing your abdominal muscles, lower back, hamstring, and buttock muscles.
- To make the exercise more challenging, hold a dumbbell between the arches of your feet and perform the exercise for the desired number of repetitions.

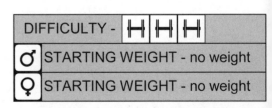

DIFFICULTY -	H H H
♂ STARTING WEIGHT - no weight	
♀ STARTING WEIGHT - no weight	

BALL STRAIGHT LEG EXTENSIONS

MAJOR MUSCLES IN USE:

Biceps Femoris, Semitendinosus, Semimembranosus, Gluteus Maximus, Adductor Magnus, Erector Spinae

STARTING POSITION:

- Position your hips slightly back from the middle top portion of an exercise ball that is balanced on the edge of an exercise bench.
- Steady your upper body by grasping on either side of the bench. Do not take your feet off the ground until you have control of your balance.
- Roll forwards slightly on the ball so that your feet are not touching the floor and your legs are hanging towards the floor. Your body should be positioned on the ball so that it is bent at 90°.
- Tense the abdominal and lower back muscles. You may wish to hold a dumbbell between your feet for added resistance.

EXERCISE MOVEMENT:

- Begin the movement by raising your straightened legs.
- Finish the exercise movement with your legs as high as possible.
- Lower your legs back to the starting position in the same arc that they were raised.

EXERCISE TECHNIQUE POINTS:

- Do not swing or bounce in the bottom position.
- Do not allow your legs to bend at any point in the motion.
- Your back should keep its normal spinal curves while doing the movement.
- Make sure you keep your back straight by tensing your abdominals, lower back, hamstring, and buttock muscles.

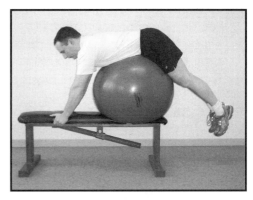

START

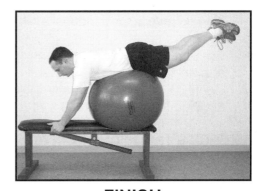

FINISH

DIFFICULTY -	H H H H H
♂	STARTING WEIGHT - no weight
♀	STARTING WEIGHT - no weight

BALL SWIMMERS

MAJOR MUSCLES IN USE:
Erector Spinae, Biceps Femoris, Semitendinosus, Gluteus Maximus

STARTING POSITION:
- Position your hips and lower mid-section on the top portion of an exercise ball.
- Place both hands and feet on the floor so that your body is bent over top of the ball.
- Tense the abdominal and lower back muscles.

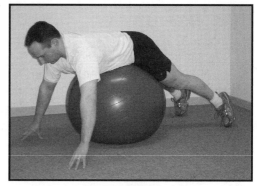

START

EXERCISE MOVEMENT:
- Begin the movement by slowly raising one arm in combination with your opposite leg. Continue to raise your arm and leg together as high as possible. Keep your shoulders and hips level with the floor by tensing your abdominal muscles.
- Once you can not raise your arm and leg any higher, reverse the motion back to the starting position.
- Perform the same movement on the opposite arm and leg.
- Continue to alternate sides until you have reached the desired number of repetitions.

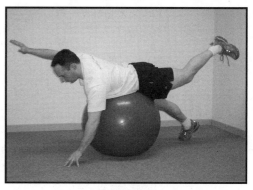

FINISH

EXERCISE TECHNIQUE POINTS:
- Make sure that you do not allow your body to twist as you raise your arm and leg by tensing your abdominal, lower back, hamstring, and buttock muscles.
- Do not allow you legs or arms to bend as your raise them.
- Do not bounce in the bottom position.
- You may wish to add a weight to each limb by by using wrist and ankle weights if you find the movement to easy.

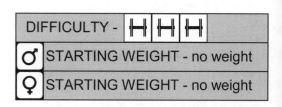

DIFFICULTY -	H H H
♂	STARTING WEIGHT - no weight
♀	STARTING WEIGHT - no weight

CHEST EXERCISES

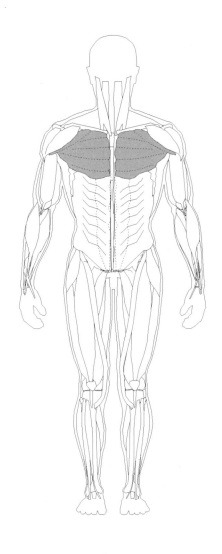

BENCH PRESS

MAJOR MUSCLES IN USE:
Pectoralis Major, Anterior Deltoid, Medial Deltoid, Triceps Brachii, Serratus Anterior

STARTING POSITION:
- Lie flat on a bench press bench and position yourself so that your eyes are directly below the bar.
- Use an overhand grip about 3 to 4 inches wider than shoulder-width.
- With your feet flat on the floor lift the bar off the uprights and position it directly above your shoulders. Your arms should be straight up so that your wrists, elbows and shoulders are supporting the weight.

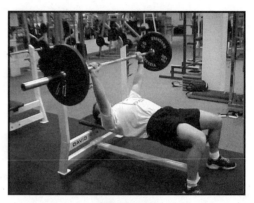

START

EXERCISE MOVEMENT:
- Lower the bar down to the middle of your chest in a very slight arc that follows the natural movement pattern of your shoulders.
- Your elbows should be pointing out to the sides to allow the chest muscles to do the majority of the work.
- Let the barbell lightly touch your chest and then push it back up following the same path in which you lowered it. At the bottom part of the movement, your forearms should be perpendicular to the floor.

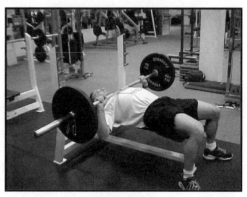

FINISH

EXERCISE TECHNIQUE POINTS:
- Do not bounce the barbell off your chest.
- Do not allow your midsection to rise off the bench since this would result in excessive arching of your back.
- Your feet should remain on the floor and your hips and lower back should remain on the bench.
- Make sure you do not allow the bar to twist (one side closer to your feet and one side closer to your head) as this could lead to shoulder problems.

DIFFICULTY -	⊢⊣ ⊦
♂ STARTING WEIGHT - 65	
♀ STARTING WEIGHT - 35	

BALL BENCH PRESS

MAJOR MUSCLES IN USE:
Pectoralis Major, Anterior Deltoid, Medial Deltoid, Triceps Brachii, Serratus Anterior

STARTING POSITION:
- Position your upper back and shoulders across the top of an exercise ball. Your feet should be flat on the floor and your hips, knees and shoulders should be in a straight line that is parallel to the floor.
- Use an overhand grip about 3 to 4 inches wider than shoulder-width.
- Lift the bar off the uprights and position it directly above your shoulders. Your arms should be straight up so that your wrists, elbows and shoulders are supporting the weight. Keep your abdominal and lower back muscles tensed to help you balance on the ball.

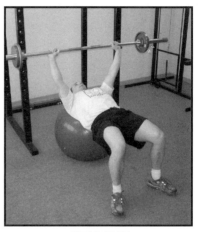

START

EXERCISE MOVEMENT:
- Lower the bar down to the middle of your chest in a very slight arc that follows the natural movement pattern of your shoulders.
- Your elbows should be pointing out to the sides to allow the chest muscles to do the majority of the work.
- Let the barbell lightly touch your chest and then push it back up following the same path in which you lowered it. At the bottom part of the movement, your forearms should be perpendicular to the floor.

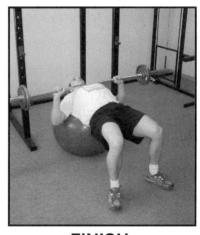

FINISH

EXERCISE TECHNIQUE POINTS:
- Do not bounce the barbell off your chest.
- Do not allow your midsection to rise higher than your hips since this would result in excessive arching of your back and an unstable position on the ball.
- Keep your abdominal and lower back muscle tensed and feet firmly planted on the floor at all times.
- Make sure you do not allow the bar to twist (one side closer to your feet and one side closer to your head) as this could lead to shoulder problems.

DIFFICULTY -	⊢⊣ ⊢
♂	STARTING WEIGHT - 55
♀	STARTING WEIGHT - 25

INCLINE BENCH PRESS

MAJOR MUSCLES IN USE:
Pectoralis Major, Anterior Deltoid, Medial Deltoid, Triceps Brachii, Serratus Anterior

STARTING POSITION:
- Lie on an incline bench and adjust the seat so that your eyes are positioned right below the bar.
- Grasp the bar with an overhand grip. Your hands should be about 3 – 4 inches wider than the width of your shoulders.
- With your feet flat on the floor, lift the bar off the uprights and position it right above your shoulders. Your arms should be straight up so that your wrists, elbows, and shoulders are in a line supporting the weight.

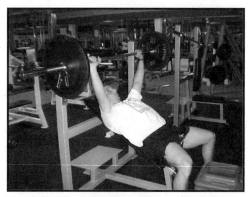

START

EXERCISE MOVEMENT:
- Lower the bar down to your upper chest so that it follows the natural movement pattern of your shoulders. Unlike the bench press exercise, there is hardly any arc to lowering this movement.
- Your elbows should be pointing out to the sides to allow the chest muscles to do the majority of the work.
- Let the barbell lightly touch your upper chest and then push it back up following the same path that you used when lowering it. At the bottom part of the repetition, your forearms should be perpendicular to the floor.

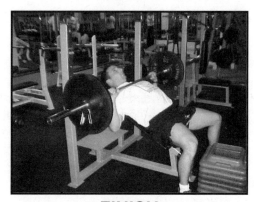

FINISH

EXERCISE TECHNIQUE POINTS:
- Do not bounce the barbell off your chest.
- Do not allow your chest to rise causing excessive arching in your lower back.
- Your feet should remain on the floor and your hips and lower back should remain on the bench.
- Make sure you do not allow the bar to twist (one side closer to your feet and one side closer to your head) as this could lead to shoulder problems.

DIFFICULTY - ┣┫ ┠	
♂	STARTING WEIGHT - 60
♀	STARTING WEIGHT - 35

CHEST EXERCISES 152

DECLINE BENCH PRESS

MAJOR MUSCLES IN USE:
Pectoralis Major, Anterior Deltoid, Medial Deltoid, Triceps Brachii, Serratus Anterior

STARTING POSITION:
- Lie on a decline bench, and adjust the leg attachment (if applicable) so that your eyes are right below the bar when it is resting on the uprights.
- Grasp the bar with an overhand grip about 3 – 4 inches wider than the width of your shoulders.
- With your feet locked under the leg attachment, lift the bar off the uprights and position it right above your shoulders. Your arms should be straight up so that your wrists, elbows, and shoulders are all in line supporting the weight.

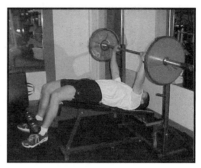

START

EXERCISE MOVEMENT:
- Lower the bar down to your lower chest so that it follows the natural movement pattern of your shoulders. Unlike the bench press exercise, there is hardly any arc to this lowering movement.
- Your elbows should be pointing out to the sides to allow the chest muscles to do the majority of the work.
- Let the barbell lightly touch your lower chest and then push it back up following the same path as when you lowered it. At the bottom part of the repetition, your forearms should be perpendicular to the floor.

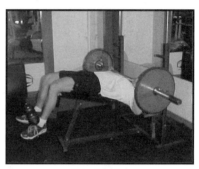

FINISH

EXERCISE TECHNIQUE POINTS:
- Do not bounce the barbell off your chest.
- Do not allow your mid-section to rise up causing excessive arching in your back.
- Make sure you do not allow the bar to twist (one side closer to your feet and one side closer to your head) as this could lead to shoulder problems.

DIFFICULTY -	⊢⊣ ⊢⊣	
♂	STARTING WEIGHT - 65	
♀	STARTING WEIGHT - 35	

CHEST EXERCISES 153

FLAT DUMBBELL PRESS

MAJOR MUSCLES IN USE:
Pectoralis Major, Anterior Deltoid, Medial Deltoid, Triceps Brachii, Serratus Anterior

STARTING POSITION:
- Lie flat on an exercise bench. Position yourself with your feet flat on the floor and your head on the bench.
- Position a pair of dumbbells straight above you with your palms facing your feet.
- Your arms should be straight so that your wrists, elbows, and shoulders are all in line. The ends of the dumbbells should be 1 – 2 inches apart.

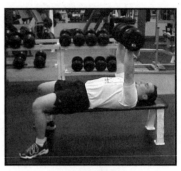

START

EXERCISE MOVEMENT:
- Lower the dumbbells down to each side of your shoulders.
- At the bottom portion of the movement your forearms should be perpendicular to the floor with your hands at the level of your shoulders and mid-chest.
- Your elbows should be pointing straight out to the sides to allow the chest muscles to do the majority of the work.
- Reverse the motion by pushing the dumbbells back along the same path that they were lowered. The dumbbells should follow a triangular path with the dumbbells farther apart at the bottom of the movement than at the top.

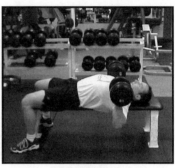

FINISH

EXERCISE TECHNIQUE POINTS:
- Do not bounce the dumbbells at the bottom of the movement.
- Do not twist the dumbbells as you are lifting them.
- Make sure that the dumbbells are positioned so that your wrists are directly above your elbows at all times.

DIFFICULTY -	H	H
♂ STARTING WEIGHT - 25		
♀ STARTING WEIGHT - 12		

BALL FLAT DUMBBELL PRESS

MAJOR MUSCLES IN USE:
Pectoralis Major, Anterior Deltoid, Medial Deltoid, Triceps Brachii, Serratus Anterior

STARTING POSITION:
- Position your upper back and shoulders across the top of an exercise ball. Your feet should be flat on the floor with your hips, knees, and shoulders in a straight line that is parallel to the floor.
- Position a pair of dumbbells straight above you with your palms facing your feet.
- Your arms should be straight so that your wrists, elbows, and shoulders are all in line. The ends of the dumbbells should be 1 – 2 inches apart.

EXERCISE MOVEMENT:
- Lower the dumbbells down to each side of your shoulders.
- At the bottom portion of the movement your forearms should be perpendicular to the floor with your hands at the level of your shoulders and mid-chest.
- Your elbows should be pointing straight out to the sides to allow the chest muscles to do the majority of the work.
- Reverse the motion by pushing the dumbbells back along the same path that they were lowered. The dumbbells should follow a triangular path with the dumbbells farther apart at the bottom of the movement than at the top.

EXERCISE TECHNIQUE POINTS:
- Do not bounce the dumbbells at the bottom of the movement.
- Do not twist the dumbbells as you are lifting them.
- Keep your abdominal and lower back muscles tensed to help you balance on the ball.
- Make sure that the dumbbells are positioned so that your wrists are directly above your elbows at all times.
- You may also choose a parallel grip where the palms of your hands face each other.

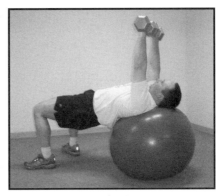
START

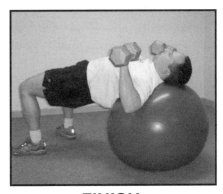
FINISH

DIFFICULTY -	H	H
♂ STARTING WEIGHT - 25		
♀ STARTING WEIGHT - 10		

CHEST EXERCISES

PARALLEL GRIP FLAT DUMBBELL PRESS

MAJOR MUSCLES IN USE:

Pectoralis Major, Anterior Deltoid, Medial Deltoid, Triceps Brachii, Serratus Anterior

STARTING POSITION:

- Lie flat on an exercise bench. Position yourself with your feet flat on the floor and your head on the bench.
- Position a pair of dumbbells straight above you with your palms facing towards each other.
- Your arms should be straight so that your wrists, elbows, and shoulders are all in line. The ends of the dumbbells should be 1 – 2 inches apart.

EXERCISE MOVEMENT:

- Lower the dumbbells down to each side of your shoulders.
- At the bottom portion of the movement your forearms should be perpendicular to the floor with your hands at the level of your shoulders and mid-chest.
- Your elbows should be pointing straight out to the sides to allow the chest muscles to do the majority of the work.
- Reverse the motion by pushing the dumbbells back along the same path that they were lowered. The dumbbells should follow a triangular path with the dumbbells farther apart at the bottom of the movement than at the top.

EXERCISE TECHNIQUE POINTS:

- Do not bounce the dumbbells at the bottom of the movement.
- Do not twist the dumbbells as you are lifting them.
- Make sure that the dumbbells are positioned so that your wrists are directly above your elbows at all times.

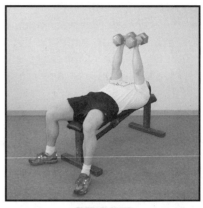

START

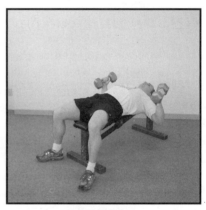

FINISH

DIFFICULTY -	H H	
♂	STARTING WEIGHT - 25	
♀	STARTING WEIGHT - 12	

CHEST EXERCISES 156

INCLINE DUMBBELL PRESS

MAJOR MUSCLES IN USE:
Pectoralis Major, Anterior Deltoid, Medial Deltoid, Triceps Brachii, Serratus Anterior

STARTING POSITION:
- Lie on an exercise bench adjusted to an angle of approximately 30° - 40° with your feet flat on the floor.
- Position a pair of dumbbells straight above you with your palms facing towards your feet.
- Your arms should be straight up so that your wrists, elbows, and shoulders are all in line. The ends of the dumbbells should be 1 – 2 inches apart.

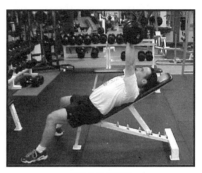

START

EXERCISE MOVEMENT:
- Lower the dumbbells down to each side of your shoulders.
- At the bottom portion of the movement your forearms should be perpendicular to the floor with your hands at the level of your shoulders and mid-chest.
- Your elbows should be pointing straight out to the sides to allow the chest muscles to do the majority of the work.
- Reverse the motion by pushing the dumbbells back along the same path that they were lowered. The dumbbells should follow a triangular path with the dumbbells farther apart at the bottom of the movement than at the top.

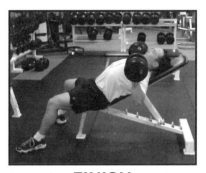

FINISH

EXERCISE TECHNIQUE POINTS:
- Do not bounce the dumbbells at the bottom of the movement.
- Do not twist the dumbbells as you are lifting them.
- Make sure that the dumbbells are always positioned so that your wrists are directly above your elbows.
- Do not allow your lower back to arch excessively when completing a repetition.

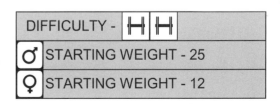

DIFFICULTY -	⊢⊣ ⊢⊣	
♂	STARTING WEIGHT - 25	
♀	STARTING WEIGHT - 12	

CHEST EXERCISES 157

INCLINE PARALLEL GRIP DUMBBELL PRESS

MAJOR MUSCLES IN USE:
Pectoralis Major, Anterior Deltoid, Medial Deltoid, Triceps Brachii, Serratus Anterior

STARTING POSITION:
- Lie on an exercise bench adjusted to an angle of approximately 30° - 40° with your feet flat on the floor.
- Position a pair of dumbbells straight above you with your palms facing towards your feet.
- Your arms should be straight up so that your wrists, elbows, and shoulders are all in line. The ends of the dumbbells should be 1 – 2 inches apart.

EXERCISE MOVEMENT:
- Lower the dumbbells down to each side of your shoulders.
- At the bottom portion of the movement your forearms should be perpendicular to the floor with your hands at the level of your shoulders and mid-chest.
- Your elbows should be pointing straight out to the sides to allow the chest muscles to do the majority of the work.
- Reverse the motion by pushing the dumbbells back along the same path that they were lowered.
- The dumbbells should follow a triangular path with the dumbbells farther apart at the bottom of the movement than at the top.

EXERCISE TECHNIQUE POINTS:
- Do not bounce the dumbbells at the bottom of the movement.
- Do not twist the dumbbells as you are lifting them.
- Make sure that the dumbbells are always positioned so that your wrists are directly above your elbows.
- Do not allow your lower back to arch excessively when completing a repetition.

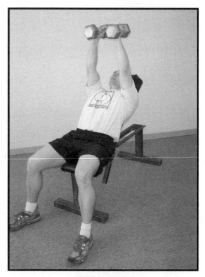

START

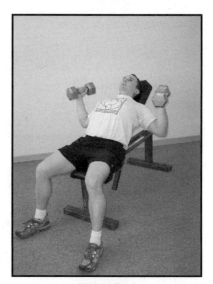

FINISH

DIFFICULTY -	H	H
♂ STARTING WEIGHT - 25		
♀ STARTING WEIGHT - 12		

DECLINE DUMBBELL PRESS

MAJOR MUSCLES IN USE:
Pectoralis Major, Anterior Deltoid, Medial Deltoid, Triceps Brachii, Serratus Anterior

STARTING POSITION:
- Lie on an exercise bench positioned at a slight decline with your feet securely anchored.
- Position a pair of dumbbells straight above you with your palms facing towards your feet.
- Your arms should be straight up so that your wrists, elbows, and shoulders are all in line. The ends of the dumbbells should be 1 – 2 inches apart.

EXERCISE MOVEMENT:
- Lower the dumbbells down to each side of your shoulders.
- At the bottom portion of the movement your forearms should be perpendicular to the floor with your hands level with your shoulders and mid-chest.
- Your elbows should be pointing straight out to the sides to allow the chest muscles to do the majority of the work.
- Reverse the motion by pushing the dumbbells back along the same path that they were lowered. The dumbbells should follow a triangular path with the dumbbells farther apart at the bottom of the movement than at the top.

EXERCISE TECHNIQUE POINTS:
- Do not bounce the dumbbells at the bottom of the movement.
- Do not twist the dumbbells as you are lifting them.
- Make sure that the dumbbells are positioned so that your wrists are always right above your elbows.
- Do not allow your lower back to arch excessively in order to complete a repetition.

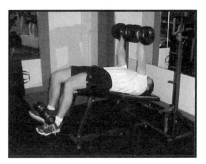

START

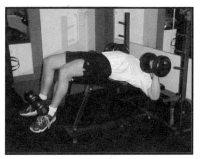

FINISH

DIFFICULTY -	H H	
♂	STARTING WEIGHT - 25	
♀	STARTING WEIGHT - 12	

CHEST EXERCISES

DECLINE PARALLEL GRIP DUMBBELL PRESS

MAJOR MUSCLES IN USE:
Pectoralis Major, Anterior Deltoid, Medial Deltoid, Triceps Brachii, Serratus Anterior

STARTING POSITION:
- Lie on an exercise bench positioned at a slight decline with your feet securely anchored.
- Position a pair of dumbbells straight above you with your palms facing each other.
- Your arms should be straight up so that your wrists, elbows, and shoulders are all in line. The ends of the dumbbells should be 1 – 2 inches apart.

EXERCISE MOVEMENT:
- Lower the dumbbells down to each side of your shoulders.
- At the bottom portion of the movement your forearms should be perpendicular to the floor with your hands level with your shoulders and mid-chest.
- Your elbows should be pointing straight out to the sides to allow the chest muscles to do the majority of the work.
- Reverse the motion by pushing the dumbbells back along the same path that they were lowered. The dumbbells should follow a triangular path with the dumbbells farther apart at the bottom of the movement than at the top.

EXERCISE TECHNIQUE POINTS:
- Do not bounce the dumbbells at the bottom of the movement.
- Do not twist the dumbbells as you are lifting them.
- Make sure that the dumbbells are positioned so that your wrists are always right above your elbows.
- Do not allow your lower back to arch excessively in order to complete a repetition.

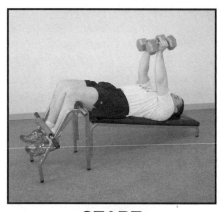

START

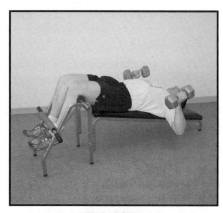

FINISH

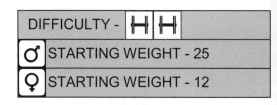

DIFFICULTY -	⊢	⊢
♂ STARTING WEIGHT - 25		
♀ STARTING WEIGHT - 12		

DUMBBELL FLAT FLY

MAJOR MUSCLES IN USE:
Pectoralis Major, Anterior Deltoid, Biceps Brachii

STARTING POSITION:
- Lie flat on an exercise bench with your feet flat on the floor.
- Arms are positioned vertically with the dumbbells centred over the neck.
- Elbows are slightly bent with palms facing each other.

EXERCISE MOVEMENT:
- While keeping your elbows always slightly bent, begin by moving the dumbbells outwards along a semicircular path that is perpendicular to your torso.
- At the end-point in the movement, the dumbbells should be level with your shoulders and your elbows should be lower than your shoulders.
- Your chest should be slightly raised and your back arched in order to keep your chest muscles in an optimal contraction position. Remember to keep your elbows slightly bent and your hands parallel to the floor.
- Finish the exercise by returning the dumbbells to the starting position in the same motion that they were lowered.

EXERCISE TECHNIQUE POINTS:
- Do not bounce the dumbbells in the bottom portion of this movement.
- Do not allow your elbows to either straighten or bend by more than 10°.
- Do not twist the dumbbells at the top of the motion.

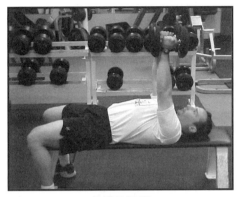

START

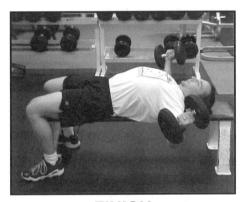

FINISH

DIFFICULTY -	⊢ ⊢ ⊢	
♂	STARTING WEIGHT - 15	
♀	STARTING WEIGHT - 8	

CHEST EXERCISES

BALL DUMBBELL FLAT FLY

MAJOR MUSCLES IN USE:
Pectoralis Major, Anterior Deltoid, Biceps Brachii

STARTING POSITION:
- Position your upper back and shoulders across the top of an exercise ball. Your feet should be flat on the floor and your hips, knees, and shoulders should be in a straight line, parallel to the floor.
- Arms are positioned vertically with the dumbbells centred over the neck.
- Elbows are slightly bent with palms facing each other.

EXERCISE MOVEMENT:
- While keeping your elbows always slightly bent, begin by moving the dumbbells outwards along a semicircular path that is perpendicular to your torso.
- At the end-point in the movement, the dumbbells should be about level with your shoulders and your elbows should be lower than your shoulders. Your chest should be slightly raised and your back arched in order to keep your chest muscles in an optimal contraction position. Remember to keep your elbows slightly bent and your hands parallel to the floor.
- Finish the exercise by returning the dumbbells to the starting position in the same motion that they were lowered.

EXERCISE TECHNIQUE POINTS:
- Do not bounce the dumbbells in the bottom portion of this movement.
- Do not allow your elbows to either straighten or bend by more than 10°.
- Do not twist the dumbbells at the top of the motion.

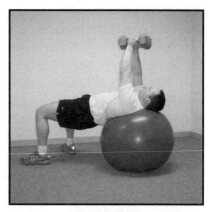
START

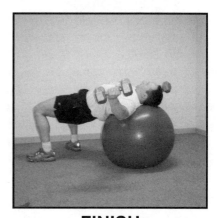
FINISH

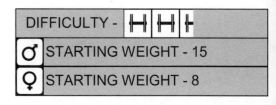

DIFFICULTY -

♂ STARTING WEIGHT - 15

♀ STARTING WEIGHT - 8

DUMBBELL INCLINE FLY

MAJOR MUSCLES IN USE:
Pectoralis Major, Anterior Deltoid, Biceps Brachii

STARTING POSITION:
- Lie on an exercise bench adjusted to approximately 30° - 40° with feet flat on the floor.
- Arms should be straight with dumbbells centred over the face.
- Elbows should be slightly bent with palms facing each other.

EXERCISE MOVEMENT:
- While always keeping your elbows slightly bent, begin by moving the dumbbells outwards along a semicircular path perpendicular to your torso.
- At the end-point in the movement, the dumbbells should be about level with your shoulders and your elbows should be lower than your shoulders. Your chest should be slightly raised and your back arched. Remember to keep your elbows slightly bent and your hands held almost parallel to the floor.
- Finish the exercise by returning the dumbbells to the starting position along the same path that they were lowered.

EXERCISE TECHNIQUE POINTS:
- Do not bounce the dumbbells in the bottom portion of this movement.
- Do not allow your elbows to either straighten or bend by more than 10°.
- Do not twist the dumbbells at the top of the motion.

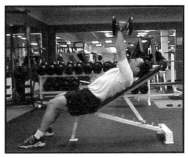

START

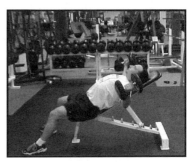

FINISH

DIFFICULTY -	H	H	H
♂ STARTING WEIGHT - 15			
♀ STARTING WEIGHT - 8			

CHEST EXERCISES

DUMBBELL DECLINE FLY

MAJOR MUSCLES IN USE:
Pectoralis Major, Anterior Deltoid, Biceps Brachii

STARTING POSITION:
- Lie on an exercise bench declined approximately 10°-20° to the floor with your feet securely anchored.
- Arms are straight with dumbbells centred over the chest.
- Elbows are slightly bent with palms facing each other.

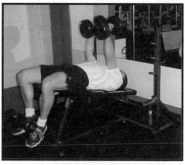

START

EXERCISE MOVEMENT:
- While keeping your elbows slightly bent, begin by moving the dumbbells outwards along an arc perpendicular to your torso.
- At the end-point in the movement, the dumbbells should be level with your chest and your elbows lower than your shoulders. Your chest should be slightly raised upwards in order to keep your chest muscles in an optimal contraction position. Remember to keep your elbows slightly bent and your hands almost parallel to the floor.
- Finish the exercise by returning the dumbbells to the starting position with the same motion that they were lowered.

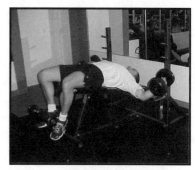

FINISH

EXERCISE TECHNIQUE POINTS:
- Do not bounce the dumbbells in the bottom portion of the movement.
- Do not allow your elbows to either straighten or bend more than 10°.
- Do not twist the dumbbells at the top of the motion.

DIFFICULTY -	H H H
♂ STARTING WEIGHT - 15	
♀ STARTING WEIGHT - 8	

CABLE CROSS-OVER

MAJOR MUSCLES IN USE:
Pectoralis Major, Anterior Deltoid, Biceps Brachii

STARTING POSITION:
- This exercise requires a special cable cross-over machine or an exercise set-up of two pulldown machines facing each other.
- Grasp each single handle with the closest hand and position yourself in the middle of the two pulleys. Place one foot in front of the other and bend over at the waist so that your torso is at about 45° to the floor.
- Your arms are slightly bent and elbows should be pointing outwards towards the pulley machines. You should feel a slight stretch in your chest muscles.

EXERCISE MOVEMENT:
- Keeping your elbows slightly bent, begin the exercise by bringing the handles together in front of your body. Your hands should move together in a semicircular arc slightly less than perpendicular to your torso.
- At the end-point in the movement, the handles should be about level with the bottom of your breastbone. You should have slightly raised your chest by arching your back in order to keep your chest muscles in an optimal contraction position.
- Remember to keep your elbows slightly bent. Your arms should be at a little less than a 45° angle to the floor.
- Finish the exercise by returning the handles back to the starting position in the same semicircular motion used in lowering them.

EXERCISE TECHNIQUE POINTS:
- Remember to stay bent over with your back straight throughout the exercise.
- Do not allow your elbows to either straighten or bend more than 10°.
- Do not twist the handles during any part of the movement.

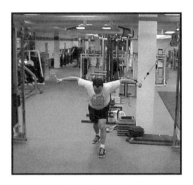

START

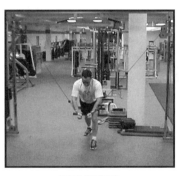

FINISH

DIFFICULTY -	H	H	H	
♂	STARTING WEIGHT - 25			
♀	STARTING WEIGHT - 10			

CABLE FLAT FLY

MAJOR MUSCLES IN USE:
Pectoralis Major, Anterior Deltoid, Biceps Brachii

STARTING POSITION:
- This exercise requires a special cable cross-over machine or an exercise set-up of two pulldown machines facing each other.
- Position the bench in the middle of the two pulleys. Grasp each handle from the low pulley of the machine. Lie flat on the exercise bench with feet flat on the floor.
- Arms should be straight up with the handles of each cable centred over the chest.
- Elbows are slightly bent with palms facing each other.

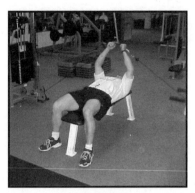

START

EXERCISE MOVEMENT:
- While keeping your elbows slightly bent, begin by moving the handles outwards in a semicircular arc perpendicular to your torso.
- At the end-point in the movement, the handles of the cables should be level with your shoulders and your elbows positioned lower than your shoulders. Your chest should also have been slightly raised by arching your back to keep your chest muscles in an optimal contraction position. Remember that to keep your elbows slightly bent, your hands should be positioned parallel to the floor.
- Finish the exercise by returning the handles to the starting position along the same semicircular motion used in lowering them.

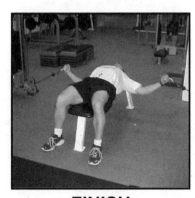

FINISH

EXERCISE TECHNIQUE POINTS:
- Do not bounce the arms in the bottom portion of this movement.
- Do not allow your elbows to either straighten or bend more than 10°.
- Do not twist the handles at the top of the motion.

DIFFICULTY -	H	H	H
♂ STARTING WEIGHT - 25			
♀ STARTING WEIGHT - 10			

BALL CABLE FLAT FLY

MAJOR MUSCLES IN USE:
Pectoralis Major, Anterior Deltoid, Biceps Brachii

STARTING POSITION:
- This exercise requires a special cable cross-over machine or an exercise set-up of two pulldown machines facing each other.
- Place an exercise ball in the middle of the two pulleys.
- Grasp each handle from the low pulley of the machine. Position your upper back and shoulders across the top of the ball. Your feet should be flat on the floor and your hips knees and shoulders should be in a straight line, parallel to the floor. Arms should be straight up with the handles of each cable centred over the chest.
- Elbows are slightly bent with palms facing each other.

EXERCISE MOVEMENT:
- While keeping your elbows slightly bent, begin by moving the handles outwards in a semicircular arc perpendicular to your torso.
- At the end-point in the movement, the handles of the cables should be level with your shoulders and your elbows positioned lower than your shoulders. Your chest should also have been slightly raised by arching your back to keep your chest muscles in an optimal contraction position. Remember that to keep your elbows slightly bent, your hands should be positioned parallel to the floor.
- Finish the exercise by returning the handles to the starting position along the same semicircular motion used in lowering them.

EXERCISE TECHNIQUE POINTS:
- Do not bounce the arms in the bottom portion of this movement.
- Do not allow your elbows to either straighten or bend more than 10°.
- Do not twist the handles at the top of the motion.

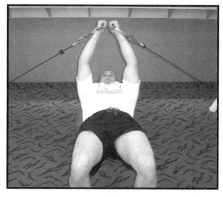

START

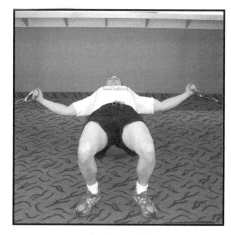

FINISH

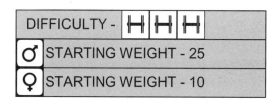

DIFFICULTY -	H	H	H
♂ STARTING WEIGHT - 25			
♀ STARTING WEIGHT - 10			

CHEST EXERCISES 167

CABLE INCLINE FLY

MAJOR MUSCLES IN USE:
Pectoralis Major, Anterior Deltoid, Biceps Brachii

STARTING POSITION:
- This exercise requires a special cable cross-over machine or an exercise set-up of two pulldown machines facing each other.
- Position the bench in the middle of the two pulleys. Grasp each handle from the low pulley of each machine. Lie on an exercise bench adjusted to approximately 30° - 40°. Your feet should be flat on the floor.
- Arms should be straight up and the handles centred over the shoulders.
- Elbows are slightly bent with palms facing each other.

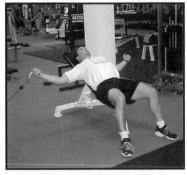

START

EXERCISE MOVEMENT:
- While keeping your elbows slightly bent, begin by moving the handles outwards in a semicircular arc while keeping your arms perpendicular to your torso.
- At the end-point in the movement, the handles should be level with your shoulders. Your elbows should be lower than your shoulders. Your chest should be slightly raised and your back arched in order to keep your chest muscles in an optimal contraction position. Remember to keep the backs of your hands almost parallel to the floor.
- Finish the exercise by returning the handles to the starting position in the same semicircular motion used in lowering them.

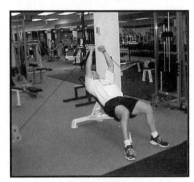

FINISH

EXERCISE TECHNIQUE POINTS:
- Do not bounce the arms in the bottom portion of this movement.
- Do not allow your elbows to either straighten or bend more than 10°.
- Do not twist the handles at the top of the motion.

DIFFICULTY -	H	H	H
♂ STARTING WEIGHT - 20			
♀ STARTING WEIGHT - 10			

CHEST EXERCISES

ONE ARM CABLE CROSS-OVER

MAJOR MUSCLES IN USE:
Pectoralis Major, Anterior Deltoid, Biceps Brachii

STARTING POSITION:
- Stand a little farther than arms-length away from the pulldown machine.
- With the hand closest to the machine, grasp the single handle from the high pulley. Place one foot in front of the other and bend over at the waist so that your torso is at 45° - 55° to the floor.
- Your arm should be slightly bent and positioned outwards in the direction of the high pulley. You should feel a slight stretch in your chest muscle.

EXERCISE MOVEMENT:
- While keeping your elbow slightly bent, begin by bringing the handle forwards in front of your body. Your hand should move in a semicircular arc slightly less than perpendicular to your torso.
- At the end-point of the movement, the handle should be in line with the bottom of your breastbone and slightly pass the midpoint of your body. Your chest should be slightly raised and your back arched in order to keep your chest muscle in an optimal contraction position.
- Remember that your elbow should be slightly bent and that your arm should be a bit less than 45° to the floor.
- Finish the exercise by returning the handle back to the starting position in the same semicircular motion used in lowering it.

EXERCISE TECHNIQUE POINTS:
- Remember to stay bent over with your back straight.
- Do not allow your elbow to either straighten or bend more than 10°.
- Do not twist the handle during any part of the movement.

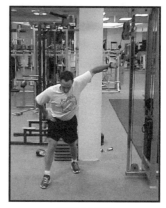

START

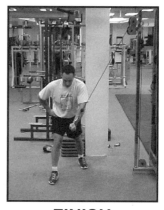

FINISH

DIFFICULTY -	H	H	H
♂ STARTING WEIGHT - 25			
♀ STARTING WEIGHT - 10			

CHEST EXERCISES 169

CHEST DIPS

MAJOR MUSCLES IN USE:
Pectoralis Major, Anterior Deltoid, Triceps Brachii

STARTING POSITION:
- Support yourself on the parallel bars of the dip station by gripping the bars with your palms facing each other. Lock your arms to support your weight.
- Angle your torso forward by extending your legs and your hips to the rear.. In order to work the chest muscles, the elbows should be out to the sides and pointing away from your body. It may be necessary for you to bend your knees at 90° so that your feet will clear the floor.

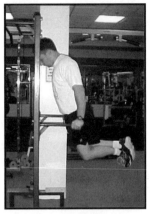

START

EXERCISE MOVEMENT:
- While keeping your upper body angled forward, descend into the bottom of the motion so that your upper arms become parallel to the floor. You should feel a stretch in the chest and shoulder muscles.
- Once your upper arms are parallel to the floor, immediately reverse the motion and push yourself back to the starting position. It is important not to pause at the bottom point of the movement.

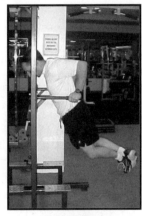

FINISH

EXERCISE TECHNIQUE POINTS:
- Remember to lean forward throughout the entire exercise.
- Keep your elbows pointed out to the sides as this will help work the chest muscles more and the triceps less.
- Do not bounce at the bottom of the movement.
- Keep your elbows parallel to the floor as much as possible in order to prevent undesirable stress on your elbows.

DIFFICULTY -	⊢ ⊢	
♂	STARTING WEIGHT – no weight	
♀	STARTING WEIGHT – no weight	

BENCH PUSHES

MAJOR MUSCLES IN USE:
Pectoralis Major, Serratus Anterior

STARTING POSITION:
- Lie on a bench press bench and position yourself so that your eyes are right below the bar.
- Use an overhand grip with hands about shoulder width apart.
- Keeping your feet flat on the floor, lift the bar off the uprights and position it right above your shoulders. Your arms should be straight up so that your wrists, elbows, and shoulders are all in line.

EXERCISE MOVEMENT:
- While keeping your arms straight and locked at the elbows, lift your shoulders off the bench as high as you can.
- When you cannot raise your shoulders any higher, lower them slowly back to the bench.

EXERCISE TECHNIQUE POINTS:
- Do not allow your elbows to bend.
- Do not allow your chest to rise up since this will result in excessive arching in your lower back.
- Your feet should remain on the floor and your hips and lower back should remain on the bench.

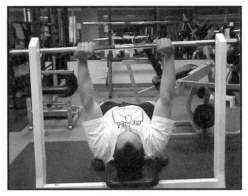

START

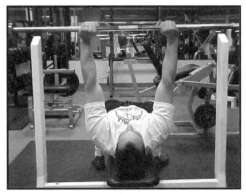

FINISH

DIFFICULTY -	⊢⊣ ⊢⊣	
♂	STARTING WEIGHT - 65	
♀	STARTING WEIGHT - 35	

CHEST EXERCISES

FRONT SHOULDER EXERCISES

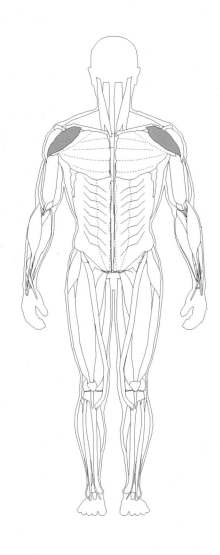

FRONT RAISES

MAJOR MUSCLES IN USE:
Anterior Deltoid, Medial Deltoid, Upper Portion of Pectoralis Major

STARTING POSITION:
- Stand with knees slightly bent.
- Hold a dumbbell in each hand and position them directly in front of your thighs.
- Elbows are to be slightly bent with palms facing towards your thighs.

EXERCISE MOVEMENT:
- Keeping your elbows slightly bent, begin by lifting one of the dumbbells forwards and away from your thigh in a semicircular arc. Your arm should travel along a path in line with the front of your body and just to the side of the midline of your torso.
- At the end point in the movement, the bar on the dumbbell should be above the level of your eyes.
- As you raise the dumbbell your palm should always be facing the floor.
- Finish the exercise by returning the dumbbell to the starting position in the same semicircular motion used in raising it.
- Repeat the exercise using the other arm.

EXERCISE TECHNIQUE POINTS:
- Do not bounce the dumbbell off your thigh in order to complete the necessary repetitions.
- Do not allow your elbow to either straighten or bend more than 10°.
- Do not allow the dumbbell to twist excessively, especially at the top of the motion.

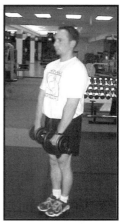

START

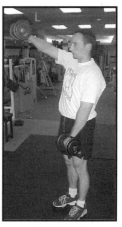

FINISH

DIFFICULTY -	H	H
♂ STARTING WEIGHT - 15		
♀ STARTING WEIGHT - 8		

HAMMER FRONT RAISES

MAJOR MUSCLES IN USE:
Anterior Deltoid, Medial Deltoid, Upper Portion of Pectoralis Major

STARTING POSITION:
- Stand with knees slightly bent and a dumbbell in each hand.
- Dumbbells should be positioned right beside your thighs.
- Elbows are slightly bent with palms facing each other.

EXERCISE MOVEMENT:
- While keeping your elbows slightly bent, begin by lifting one of the dumbbells forward and away from your thigh in a semicircular arc. Your arm should travel a path in line with the front of your body, just to the side of the midline of your torso.
- At the end point in the movement, your wrist should be about level with your eyes.
- As you raise the dumbbell, your palm should always be perpendicular to the floor.
- Finish the exercise by returning the dumbbell to the starting position following the same path by which you raised it.
- Repeat the exercise using the other arm.

EXERCISE TECHNIQUE POINTS:
- Do not bounce the dumbbell off your thigh in order to complete the necessary repetitions.
- Do not allow your elbow to either straighten or bend more than 10°.
- Do not allow the dumbbell to twist excessively, especially at the top of the motion.

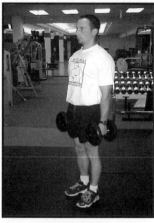

START

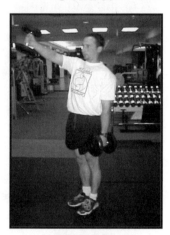

FINISH

DIFFICULTY -	⊢⊣	⊢⊣
♂ STARTING WEIGHT - 15		
♀ STARTING WEIGHT - 8		

FRONT SHOULDER EXERCISES

CABLE FRONT RAISES

MAJOR MUSCLES IN USE:
Anterior Deltoid, Medial Deltoid, Upper Portion of Pectoralis Major

STARTING POSITION:
- Stand with knees slightly bent and in front of the low pulley machine.
- Grasp the short bar attached to the low pulley with an overhand grip and straddle the cable so that it runs between your legs.
- Stand as close as you can to the pulley without interfering with the cable.
- Keep your elbows slightly bent with palms facing towards your thighs.

EXERCISE MOVEMENT:
- Keeping your elbows slightly bent, begin by lifting the bar forwards and away from your thighs in a semicircular arc. Your arms should travel upwards directly in front of your body following the midline of your torso.
- At the end point in the movement the bar should be about level with your eyes.
- Finish the exercise by lowering the bar back to the starting position using the same semicircular motion.

EXERCISE TECHNIQUE POINTS:
- Do not bounce the bar off your thighs in order to complete the necessary repetitions.
- Do not allow your elbows to either straighten or bend more than 10°.
- Be careful of the path of the cable between your legs. It may be advisable to stand on a low platform in order to give extra clearance.

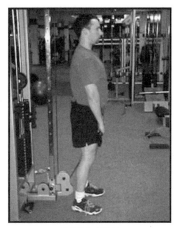

START

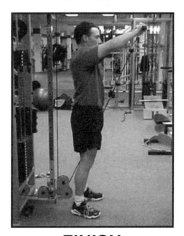

FINISH

DIFFICULTY - ⊢⊣	
♂ STARTING WEIGHT - 30	
♀ STARTING WEIGHT - 15	

ONE ARM CABLE FRONT RAISES

MAJOR MUSCLES IN USE:
Anterior Deltoid, Medial Deltoid, Upper Portion of Pectoralis Major

STARTING POSITION:
- Stand with knees slightly bent and in front of the low pulley machine.
- Facing away from the pulley machine, grasp with one hand the handle attached to the low pulley using an overhand grip. You should be standing beside the cable.
- Position the handle directly beside your upper thigh.
- Stand approximately 12 inches in front of the pulley.
- Keep your elbow slightly bent.

EXERCISE MOVEMENT:
- Begin by lifting the handle directly forwards in a semicircular arc.
- At the end point in the movement your hand should be about level with your eyes and your elbow still bent slightly.
- Finish the exercise by returning the handle back to the starting position following the same semicircular pathway used in raising it.

EXERCISE TECHNIQUE POINTS:
- Do not jerk the handle at the starting position in order to complete the necessary repetitions.
- Do not allow your elbow to either straighten or bend more than 10°.
- Be careful not to touch the cable as some cables can be abrasive or greasy.

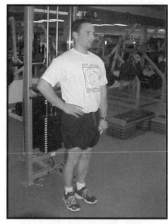

START

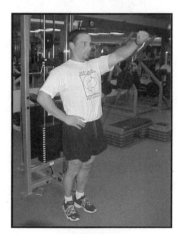

FINISH

DIFFICULTY -	H	H
♂ STARTING WEIGHT - 15		
♀ STARTING WEIGHT - 10		

OVERHEAD DUMBBELL LATERALS

MAJOR MUSCLES IN USE:
Anterior Deltoid, Medial Deltoid, Upper Portion of Pectoralis Major

STARTING POSITION:
- Stand with knees slightly bent.
- Hold the dumbbells directly above your head with your elbows slightly bent and your palms facing each other.

EXERCISE MOVEMENT:
- Keeping your elbows slightly bent and your palms facing up, lower the dumbbells directly out to your sides in a semicircular arc.
- At the end point in the movement your palms should still be facing upwards. Your hands should be level with your shoulders while your elbows remain slightly bent.
- Finish the exercise by returning the dumbbells to the starting position along the same semicircular motion.

EXERCISE TECHNIQUE POINTS:
- Do not allow your elbows to either straighten or bend more than 10°.
- Do not allow the dumbbells to twist excessively, especially at the bottom portion of the motion.
- Make sure your palms are always parallel to the floor.
- Do not allow the dumbbells to go lower than shoulder height.

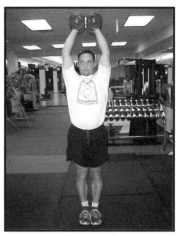

START

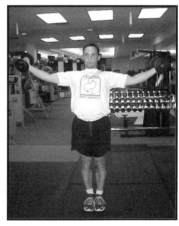

FINISH

DIFFICULTY -	⊦⊣ ⊦⊣ ⊢	
♂	STARTING WEIGHT - 10	
♀	STARTING WEIGHT - 5	

FRONT SHOULDER EXERCISES 177

ARNOLD PRESS

MAJOR MUSCLES IN USE:
Anterior Deltoid, Medial Deltoid, Upper Portion of Pectoralis Major

STARTING POSITION:
- Sit on a bench with a back support.
- Dumbbells should be positioned directly in front of and level with your shoulders.
- Elbows should be bent so that your palms are also facing towards your shoulders.

EXERCISE MOVEMENT:
- Begin the movement by raising the dumbbells and slowly rotating your palms away from your body.
- By the mid-point of the movement your palms should be facing forward, your elbows should be bent at approximately 90°, and your wrists should be directly over top of your elbows.
- At the end point in the movement your arms should be fully extended with your palms facing forward so that your wrists and elbows are positioned directly above your shoulders.

EXERCISE TECHNIQUE POINTS:
- Do not bounce the dumbbells in the bottom portion of the movement.
- If you are not using a backrest make sure you keep your abdominal muscles tensed.
- Be careful not to arch your lower back too much at the top portion of the movement.

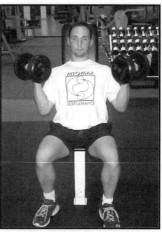

START

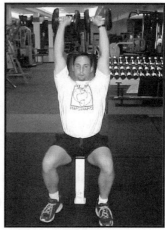

FINISH

DIFFICULTY -	H	H
♂ STARTING WEIGHT - 20		
♀ STARTING WEIGHT - 10		

DUMBBELL SHOULDER PRESS

MAJOR MUSCLES IN USE:
Anterior Deltoid, Medial Deltoid, Upper Portion of Pectoralis Major

STARTING POSITION:
- Sit on a bench with a back support.
- Dumbbells should be held at the sides of your torso and level with your shoulders.
- Elbows are bent and your palms should be positioned facing forward.

EXERCISE MOVEMENT:
- Begin the movement by raising the dumbbells upward while keeping your palms facing forward.
- By the mid-point of the movement your palms should be still facing forward, your elbows should be bent at approximately 90°, and your wrists should be directly over top of your elbows.
- At the end point in the movement your arms should be fully extended with your palms facing forward so that your wrists and elbows are positioned directly above your shoulders.

EXERCISE TECHNIQUE POINTS:
- Do not bounce the dumbbells in the bottom portion of the movement.
- If you are not using a backrest make sure to keep your abdominal muscles tensed.
- Be careful not to arch your lower back too much at the top portion of the movement.
- This exercise may also be performed standing.

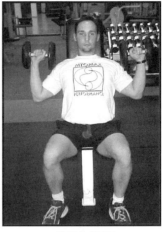

START

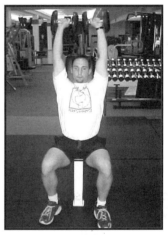

FINISH

DIFFICULTY - ⪢	
♂	STARTING WEIGHT - 20
♀	STARTING WEIGHT - 10

FRONT SHOULDER EXERCISES 179

BALL DUMBBELL SHOULDER PRESS

MAJOR MUSCLES IN USE:
Anterior Deltoid, Medial Deltoid, Upper Portion of Pectoralis Major

STARTING POSITION:
- Sit on top of an exercise ball with your feet positioned about shoulder width apart.
- Dumbbells should be held at the sides of your torso and level with your shoulders.
- Elbows are bent and your palms should be positioned facing forward.

EXERCISE MOVEMENT:
- Begin the movement by raising the dumbbells upward while keeping your palms facing forward.
- By the mid-point of the movement your palms should be still facing forward, your elbows should be bent at approximately 90°, and your wrists should be directly over top of your elbows.
- At the end point in the movement your arms should be fully extended with your palms facing forward so that your wrists and elbows are positioned directly above your shoulders.

EXERCISE TECHNIQUE POINTS:
- Do not bounce the dumbbells in the bottom portion of the movement.
- Make sure to keep your abdominal muscles tensed.
- Be careful not to arch your lower back too much at the top portion of the movement.

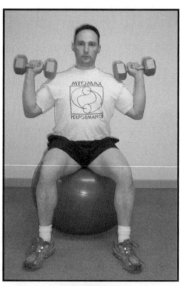

START

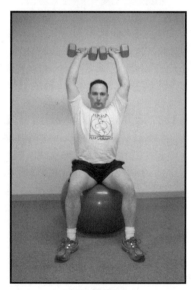

FINISH

DIFFICULTY -	⊟ ⊟	
♂	STARTING WEIGHT - 20	
♀	STARTING WEIGHT - 10	

FRONT SHOULDER EXERCISES 180

PARALLEL DUMBBELL SHOULDER PRESS

MAJOR MUSCLES IN USE:
Anterior Deltoid, Medial Deltoid, Upper Portion of Pectoralis Major

STARTING POSITION:
- Sit on a bench with a back support.
- Dumbbells should be positioned at the sides of your torso and level with your shoulders.
- Elbows are bent and your palms should face each other.
- Your arms should be placed so that your upper body resembles a "W" shape.

EXERCISE MOVEMENT:
- Begin the movement by raising the dumbbells upward while keeping your palms facing each other.
- By the mid-point of the movement your palms should still be facing each other, your elbows should be bent at approximately 90°, and your wrists should be directly over top of your elbows.
- At the end point in the movement your arms should be fully extended with your palms still facing each other so that your wrists and elbows are positioned directly above your shoulders.

EXERCISE TECHNIQUE POINTS:
- Do not bounce the dumbbells in the bottom portion of the movement.
- If you are not using a backrest make sure to keep your abdominal muscles tensed.
- Be careful not to arch your lower back too much at the top portion of the movement.
- This exercise may also be performed standing.

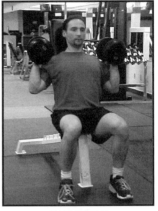

START

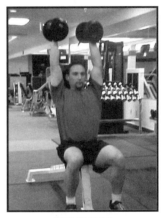

FINISH

DIFFICULTY -	⊢⊣	
♂	STARTING WEIGHT - 20	
♀	STARTING WEIGHT - 10	

ALTERNATE DUMBBELL SHOULDER PRESS

MAJOR MUSCLES IN USE:
Anterior Deltoid, Medial Deltoid, Upper Portion of Pectoralis Major

STARTING POSITION:
- Sit on a bench with a back support.
- Dumbbells should be positioned at the sides of your torso and level with your shoulders.
- Elbows are bent and your palms should face forward.
- Your arms should be placed so that your upper body resembles a "W" shape.

EXERCISE MOVEMENT:
- Begin the movement by raising one of the dumbbells upward while keeping your palms facing forward.
- By the mid-point of the movement your palms should still be facing forward, your elbow should be bent at approximately 90°, and your wrist should be directly over top of your elbow.
- At the end point in the movement your arms should be fully extended with your palms still facing forward so that your wrists and elbows are positioned directly above your shoulders.
- Lower the dumbbell back to the starting position and repeat the movement using the other arm.

EXERCISE TECHNIQUE POINTS:
- Do not bounce the dumbbells in the bottom portion of the movement.
- If you are not using a backrest make sure to keep your abdominal muscles tensed.
- Be careful not to arch your lower back too much at the top portion of the movement.
- This exercise may also be performed standing

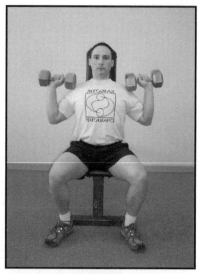

START

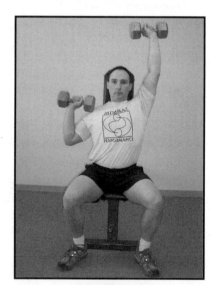

FINISH

DIFFICULTY -	H	
♂	STARTING WEIGHT - 15	
♀	STARTING WEIGHT - 8	

MILITARY PRESS

MAJOR MUSCLES IN USE:
Anterior Deltoid, Medial Deltoid, Upper Portion of Pectoralis Major

STARTING POSITION:
- Sit on a bench with a back support. In most fitness clubs there is a shoulder station specifically designed for this exercise.
- Grasp a barbell with both hands spaced shoulder width apart and palms facing forward.
- Position the barbell directly above your body with your arms fully extended.

EXERCISE MOVEMENT:
- Begin the movement by lowering the barbell down towards your upper chest.
- You should be leaning back slightly so that your head, and particularly your nose, will clear the bar as it is lowered.
- Lower the bar to the base of the neck and immediately reverse the movement so that you raise the barbell back to the starting position.

EXERCISE TECHNIQUE POINTS:
- Do not bounce the barbell at the bottom portion of the movement or off the top of the chest.
- If you are not using a backrest make sure you keep your abdominal muscles tensed and pelvis tilted slightly backwards.
- Be careful not to arch your lower back too much at any point in the movement.
- Take care that you do not strike your face with the bar while either lowering or raising the barbell.

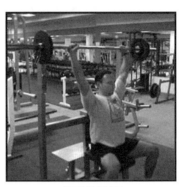

START

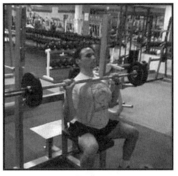

FINISH

DIFFICULTY -	⊢⊢	
♂	STARTING WEIGHT - 50	
♀	STARTING WEIGHT - 20	

PRESS BEHIND-THE-NECK

MAJOR MUSCLES IN USE:
Anterior Deltoid, Medial Deltoid, Upper Portion of Pectoralis Major

STARTING POSITION:
- Sit on a bench with a back support. In most fitness clubs there is a shoulder station specifically designed for this exercise.
- Grasp a barbell with both hands slightly more than shoulder width apart and your palms facing forward.
- Position the barbell directly above your body with your arms fully extended.

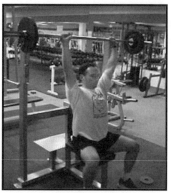
START

EXERCISE MOVEMENT:
- Begin the movement by lowering the barbell towards the upper portion of the back of your neck.
- You should be leaning forward slightly so that your head will clear the bar as it is lowered.
- Lower the bar to the middle of the back of your neck and immediately reverse the movement so that you raise the barbell back to the starting position.

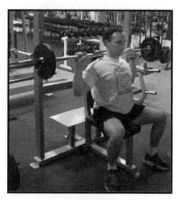
FINISH

EXERCISE TECHNIQUE POINTS:
- Do not over rotate your shoulders by bringing your elbows backwards as this can put excess stress on the shoulder muscles.
- If you are not using a backrest make sure you keep your abdominal muscles tensed and pelvis tilted slightly backwards.
- Be careful not to arch your lower back too much at any point in the movement.
- Be careful that you do not strike your neck or the back of your head with the bar while lowering or raising the barbell.
- Be careful not to lower the bar too far as this can also put excess stress on the shoulders.

DIFFICULTY -	⊢⊣ ⊢⊣ ⊢
♂ STARTING WEIGHT - 50	
♀ STARTING WEIGHT - 20	

FRONT SHOULDER EXERCISES 184

PUSH PRESS

MAJOR MUSCLES IN USE:
Anterior Deltoid, Medial Deltoid, Upper Portion of Pectoralis Major

STARTING POSITION:
- Stand with your abdominal muscles tensed.
- Grasp a barbell with hands slightly wider than shoulder width apart. Hold it at the base of the front of your neck. Your palms should now be facing forward. Often the bar is lifted directly off of a high barbell rack in order to make it easier to position the bar properly.
- One foot should be placed in front of the other to brace yourself for the exercise.

EXERCISE MOVEMENT:
- Begin the movement by slightly bending the knees and rapidly straightening them in order to gain enough momentum to begin pushing the barbell up.
- Continue to push the barbell up until your arms are fully extended and your elbows are almost locked.
- Reverse the movement by lowering the bar carefully back to the starting position.

EXERCISE TECHNIQUE POINTS:
- Do not bounce the barbell in the bottom portion of the movement or off the top of the chest. Absorb the force of the barbell by bending the knees.
- Make sure you keep your abdominal muscles tensed and pelvis tilted slightly forwards.
- Be careful not to arch your lower back too much at any point in the movement.
- Be careful that you do not strike your face with the bar while either lowering or raising the barbell.

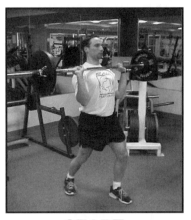

START

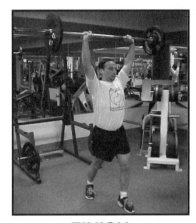

FINISH

DIFFICULTY -	⊢⊢ ⊢⊢ ⊢⊢ ⊢⊢
♂ STARTING WEIGHT - 65	
♀ STARTING WEIGHT - 35	

SHOULDER CLOSE GRIP PRESS

MAJOR MUSCLES IN USE:
Anterior Deltoid, Medial Deltoid, Pectoralis Major, Triceps, Serratus Anterior

STARTING POSITION:
- Lie on a bench press bench and position yourself so that your eyes are right below the bar.
- Use an overhand grip with hands about shoulder width apart.
- With your feet flat on the floor, lift the bar off the uprights and position it right above your shoulders. Your arms should be straight up so that your wrists, elbows, and shoulders are all in line.

EXERCISE MOVEMENT:
- Lower the bar down to the lower portion of your chest in a slight arc so that it follows the natural movement pattern of your shoulders.
- Your elbows should be kept close to your sides to allow the front shoulder and triceps muscles to do the majority of the work.
- Let the barbell lightly touch the bottom of your chest and then push it back up along the same path you used for lowering it. At the bottom part of the repetition your forearms should be nearly perpendicular to the floor.

EXERCISE TECHNIQUE POINTS:
- Do not bounce the barbell off your chest.
- Do not allow your midsection to rise up causing your lower back to arch.
- Your feet should remain on the floor and your hips and upper back should remain on the bench.
- Make sure you do not allow the bar to twist (one side closer to your feet and one side closer to your head) as this could lead to shoulder problems in the future.

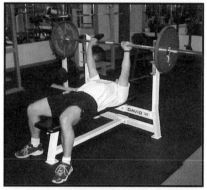

START

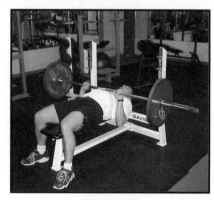

FINISH

DIFFICULTY -	H	H	
♂	STARTING WEIGHT - 55		
♀	STARTING WEIGHT - 25		

SIDE SHOULDER EXERCISES

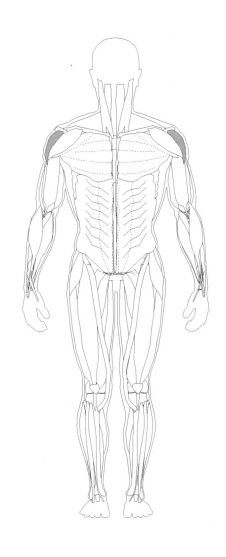

SIDE LATERALS

MAJOR MUSCLES IN USE:
Medial Deltoid, Trapezius

STARTING POSITION:
- Stand with knees slightly bent.
- Dumbbells should be held at the side of your thighs.
- Elbows should be slightly bent with palms facing towards your thighs.

EXERCISE MOVEMENT:
- While keeping your elbows slightly bent, begin by lifting the dumbbells outwards and away from your thighs in a semicircular arc. Your arms should be perpendicular to your torso.
- At the end point in the movement the bar on the dumbbell should be about level with your eyes while your elbows remain slightly bent.
- As you raise the dumbbells your palms should always be facing the floor.
- Finish the exercise by returning the dumbbells to the starting position in the same semicircular motion that they were raised.

EXERCISE TECHNIQUE POINTS:
- Do not bounce the dumbbells off your thighs in order to complete the necessary repetitions.
- Do not allow your elbows to either straighten or bend more than 10°.
- A slight twist of the dumbbells at the top of the motion so that your index finger is lower than your little finger will keep the medial deltoid in a strong contraction position.
- Do not allow your index finger to rise higher than your little finger.

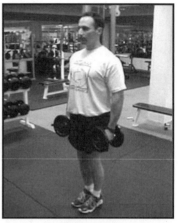

START

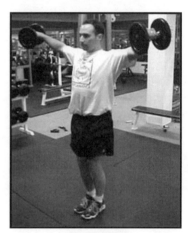

FINISH

DIFFICULTY -	⊢⊣ ⊢⊣	
♂	STARTING WEIGHT - 15	
♀	STARTING WEIGHT - 8	

SIDE SHOULDER EXERCISES 188

BALL SIDE LATERALS

MAJOR MUSCLES IN USE:
Medial Deltoid, Trapezius

STARTING POSITION:
- Sit on top of an exercise bench with both feet on the floor.
- Dumbbells should be held at your sides so that they are touching the exercise ball.
- Elbows should be slightly bent with palms facing each other.

EXERCISE MOVEMENT:
- While keeping your elbows slightly bent, begin by lifting the dumbbells outwards and away from your thighs in a semicircular arc. Your arms should be perpendicular to your torso.
- At the end point in the movement the bar on the dumbbell should be about level with your eyes while your elbows remain slightly bent.
- As you raise the dumbbells your palms should always be facing the floor.
- Finish the exercise by returning the dumbbells to the starting position in the same semicircular motion that they were raised.

EXERCISE TECHNIQUE POINTS:
- Do not bounce the dumbbells off the ball in order to complete the necessary repetitions.
- Do not allow your elbows to either straighten or bend more than 10°.
- A slight twist of the dumbbells at the top of the motion so that your index finger is lower than your little finger will keep the medial deltoid in a strong contraction position.
- Do not allow your index finger to rise higher than your little finger.
- Keep your abdominal muscles tensed to help stop your torso from rocking back and forth.
- If you find it difficult to balance try positioning your feet wider apart.

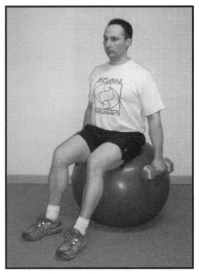

START

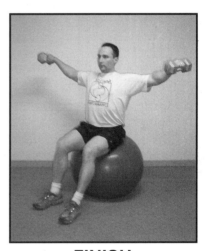

FINISH

DIFFICULTY -	⊢	⊢	
♂	STARTING WEIGHT - 15		
♀	STARTING WEIGHT - 8		

SIDE SHOULDER EXERCISES 189

SEATED SIDE LATERALS

MAJOR MUSCLES IN USE:
Medial Deltoid, Trapezius

STARTING POSITION:
- Sit on the end of an exercise bench with both feet on the floor.
- Dumbbells should be held at your sides so that they are below the exercise bench.
- Elbows should be slightly bent with palms facing each other.

EXERCISE MOVEMENT:
- While keeping your elbows slightly bent, begin by lifting the dumbbells outwards and away from your thighs in a semicircular arc. Your arms should be perpendicular to your torso.
- At the end point in the movement the bar on the dumbbell should be about level with your eyes while your elbows remain slightly bent.
- As you raise the dumbbells your palms should always be facing the floor.
- Finish the exercise by returning the dumbbells to the starting position in the same semicircular motion that they were raised.

EXERCISE TECHNIQUE POINTS:
- Do not bounce the dumbbells off your sides in order to complete the necessary repetitions.
- Do not allow your elbows to either straighten or bend more than 10°.
- A slight twist of the dumbbells at the top of the motion so that your index finger is lower than your little finger will keep the medial deltoid in a strong contraction position.
- Do not allow your index finger to rise higher than your little finger.
- Keep your abdominal muscles tensed to help stop your torso from rocking back and forth.

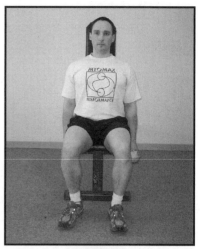

START

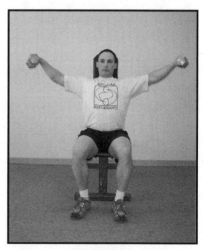

FINISH

DIFFICULTY -	H	H	
♂	STARTING WEIGHT - 10		
♀	STARTING WEIGHT - 5		

ONE ARM SIDE LATERALS

MAJOR MUSCLES IN USE:
Medial Deltoid, Trapezius

STARTING POSITION:
- Stand with your knees slightly bent.
- One dumbbell should be at the side of your thigh with your palm facing towards your thigh and your elbow slightly bent.
- Place your other hand on your hip.

EXERCISE MOVEMENT:
- While keeping your elbow slightly bent, begin by lifting the dumbbell outwards and away from your thigh in a semicircular arc. Your arm should travel along a path that is perpendicular to your torso.
- At the end point of the movement, the bar on the dumbbell should be about level with your eyes while your elbow remains slightly bent.
- As you raise the dumbbell your palm should face the floor.
- Finish the exercise by returning the dumbbell to the starting position using the same semicircular motion by which it was raised.
- Once you have completed all the repetitions for one arm, repeat the procedure for the other arm.

EXERCISE TECHNIQUE POINTS:
- Do not bounce the dumbbell off your thigh in order to complete the necessary repetitions.
- Do not allow your elbow to either straighten or bend more than 10°.
- Do not allow your index finger to rise higher than your little finger.
- A slight twist of the dumbbell at the top of the motion so that your index finger is lower than your little finger will keep the medial deltoid in a strong contraction position.
- Do not allow your torso to lean to one side in order to complete the repetition.

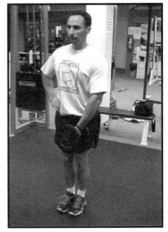

START

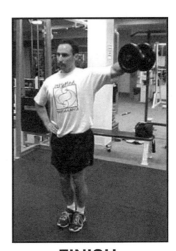

FINISH

DIFFICULTY -	H	H	
♂	STARTING WEIGHT - 15		
♀	STARTING WEIGHT - 8		

SIDE SHOULDER EXERCISES 191

SEATED ONE ARM SIDE LATERALS

MAJOR MUSCLES IN USE:
Medial Deltoid, Trapezius

STARTING POSITION:
- Sit on the end of an exercise bench with both feet on the floor.
- One dumbbell should be held at your side, below the level of the bench, with your palm facing towards your body and your elbow slightly bent.
- Your other hand should grasp the bench.

EXERCISE MOVEMENT:
- While keeping your elbow slightly bent, begin by lifting the dumbbell outwards and away from your thigh in a semicircular arc. Your arm should travel along a path that is perpendicular to your torso.
- At the end point of the movement, the bar on the dumbbell should be about level with your eyes while your elbow remains slightly bent.
- As you raise the dumbbell your palm should face the floor.
- Finish the exercise by returning the dumbbell to the starting position using the same semicircular motion by which it was raised.
- Once you have completed all the repetitions for one arm, repeat the procedure for the other arm.

EXERCISE TECHNIQUE POINTS:
- Do not bounce the dumbbell off your thigh in order to complete the necessary repetitions.
- Do not allow your elbow to either straighten or bend more than 10°.
- Do not allow your index finger to rise higher than your little finger.
- A slight twist of the dumbbell at the top of the motion so that your index finger is lower than your little finger will keep the medial deltoid in a strong contraction position.
- Do not allow your torso to lean to one side in order to complete the repetition.

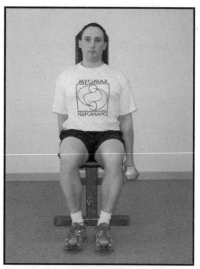

START

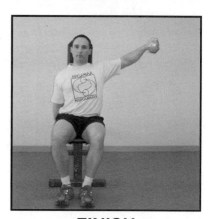

FINISH

DIFFICULTY - H H		
♂	STARTING WEIGHT - 10	
♀	STARTING WEIGHT - 5	

SIDE SHOULDER EXERCISES

CABLE SIDE LATERALS

MAJOR MUSCLES IN USE:
Medial Deltoid, Trapezius

STARTING POSITION:
- Stand in front of a low pulley with feet about shoulder width apart.
- Grasp a single handle attached to the low cable and position it directly in front of the midline of your body.
- Your elbow should be slightly bent with your palm facing to the side.

EXERCISE MOVEMENT:
- While keeping your elbow slightly bent, begin by lifting the handle outwards and away from your midline in a semicircular arc directly to the side of your torso.
- At the end point in the movement the handle should be about level with your eyes and your elbow should still be slightly bent.
- As you raise the handle, your palm should always be facing the floor.
- Finish the exercise by returning the handle to the starting position in the same semicircular motion used in raising it.

EXERCISE TECHNIQUE POINTS:
- Do not allow your torso to lean excessively to one side in order to complete the necessary repetitions.
- Do not allow your elbows to either straighten or bend more than 10°.
- Make sure that the palm of your hand faces the floor at the top portion of the exercise.
- Do not allow your index finger to rise higher than your little finger.
- Make sure that you raise your hand at least to the level of your eyes.

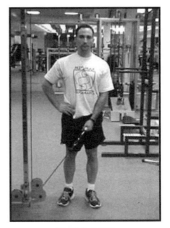

START

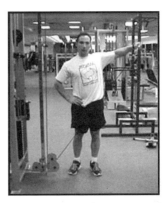

FINISH

DIFFICULTY -	�H H H
♂ STARTING WEIGHT - 15	
♀ STARTING WEIGHT - 10	

SIDE SHOULDER EXERCISES   193

INCLINE SIDE LATERALS

MAJOR MUSCLES IN USE:
Medial Deltoid, Trapezius

STARTING POSITION:
- Lie sideways on a bench at an incline of approximately 40° - 50°. Position yourself so that the front of your body is near the edge of the bench.
- With your free arm holding a dumbbell, let the dumbbell hang across the front of your body and chest so that your arm is almost hanging straight down at the side of the bench.
- Your elbow should be slightly bent with your palm positioned perpendicular to your body.

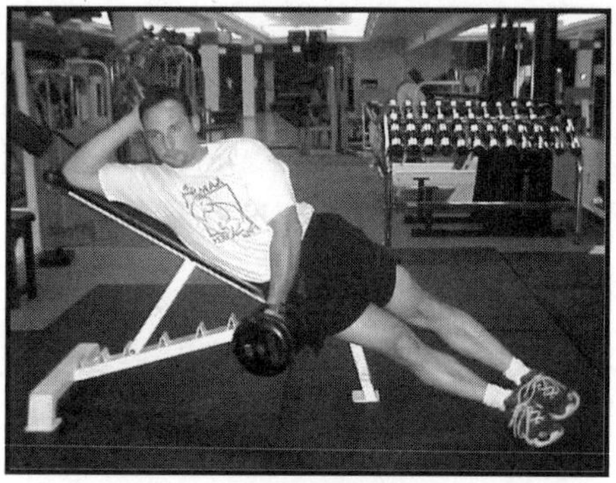

START

EXERCISE MOVEMENT:
- While keeping your elbow slightly bent, begin by lifting the dumbbell directly out to the side, allowing the dumbbell to travel upward in a semicircular arc.
- At the end-point in the movement your arm should be approximately 45° to the floor.
- As you raise the dumbbell, keep your palm facing the floor.
- Finish the exercise by returning the dumbbell to the starting position along the same semicircular path by which it was raised.

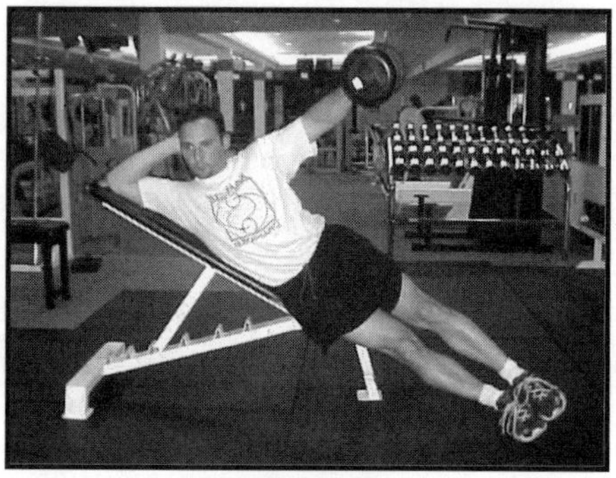

FINISH

EXERCISE TECHNIQUE POINTS:
- Do not allow your elbows to either straighten or bend more than 10°.
- Make sure that the palm of your hand faces the floor at the top portion of the exercise.
- A slight twist of the dumbbell at the top of the motion so that your index finger is lower than your little finger will keep the medial deltoid in a strong contraction position.
- Do not allow your index finger to rise higher than your little finger.

DIFFICULTY -
♂ STARTING WEIGHT - 15
♀ STARTING WEIGHT - 8

UPRIGHT ROW

MAJOR MUSCLES IN USE:
Medial Deltoid, Trapezius, Upper Portion of Pectoralis Major

STARTING POSITION:
- Stand with feet about shoulder width apart and take an over hand grip on the barbell so that your hands are placed about 6 – 8 inches apart.
- Allow your arms to straighten so that the bar hangs just above your mid-thigh.
- Bend your knees slightly and straighten your back and shoulders by keeping your chest up.

EXERCISE MOVEMENT:
- While keeping your chest high pull the bar up towards your collarbone.
- Make sure that your elbows always stay above the bar and move directly out to your sides.
- As you lift the bar, allow the bar to follow the contour of your body and stop at the base of your neck.
- Lower the bar back to the starting position along the same path that it was raised.

EXERCISE TECHNIQUE POINTS:
- Do not allow your elbows to fall below the level of the bar.
- Make sure that you hold your chest high throughout the whole movement.
- Make sure that you keep your heels on the floor.
- Do not rock your upper body back and forth in completing the necessary repetitions.

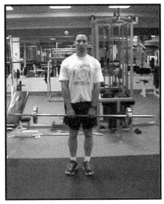

START

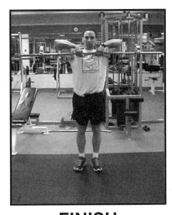

FINISH

DIFFICULTY -	⊢⊣ ⊢⊣	
♂	STARTING WEIGHT - 55	
♀	STARTING WEIGHT - 25	

SIDE SHOULDER EXERCISES

CABLE UPRIGHT ROW

MAJOR MUSCLES IN USE:
Medial Deltoid, Trapezius, Upper Portion of Pectoralis Major

STARTING POSITION:
- Standing with feet about shoulder-width apart, take an overhand grip with your hands about 6 – 8 inches apart on a short bar attached to the low pulley of a cable machine.
- Allow your arms to straighten so that the bar hangs just above your mid- thigh.
- Bend your knees slightly and straighten your back and shoulders by keeping your chest up.

EXERCISE MOVEMENT:
- While keeping your chest held high, pull the bar up towards your collarbone.
- Make sure that your elbows always stay above the bar and move directly out to the sides.
- Allow the bar to follow the contour of your body and to stop at the base of your neck.
- Lower the bar back to the starting position along the same path that it was raised.

EXERCISE TECHNIQUE POINTS:
- Do not allow your elbows to fall below the level of the bar.
- Make sure that you hold your chest high throughout the whole movement.
- Make sure that you keep your heels on the floor.
- Do not rock your torso back and forth in order to complete the necessary repetitions.
- Make sure you keep the bar close to your body at all times.

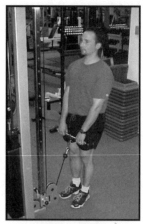

START

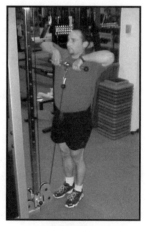

FINISH

DIFFICULTY - ┠ ┠	
♂	STARTING WEIGHT - 55
♀	STARTING WEIGHT - 25

SIDE SHOULDER EXERCISES 196

DUMBBELL UPRIGHT ROW

MAJOR MUSCLES IN USE:
Medial Deltoid, Trapezius, Upper Portion of Pectoralis Major

STARTING POSITION:
- Stand with feet about shoulder width apart and grasp each dumbbell with an overhand grip. Place your hands so that your palms are facing your legs and the dumbbells and are about 6 – 8 inches apart.
- Allow your arms to straighten so that the dumbbells hang just above your mid- thigh.
- Bend your knees slightly and straighten your back and your shoulders by keeping your chest held high.

EXERCISE MOVEMENT:
- While keeping your chest high, pull the dumbbells up towards your collarbone so that the dumbbells follow the path of a narrow "V".
- Make sure that your elbows always stay above the dumbbells and move directly out to the sides.
- Allow the dumbbells to follow the contour of your body and to stop at the base of your neck or level with you collar bone.
- Lower the dumbbells back to the starting position along the same path that they were raised.

EXERCISE TECHNIQUE POINTS:
- Do not allow your elbows to fall below the level of the dumbbells.
- Make sure that you hold your chest high throughout the whole movement.
- Make sure you keep your heels on the floor.
- Do not rock your torso back and forth in order to complete the necessary repetitions.

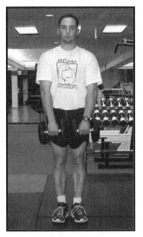

START

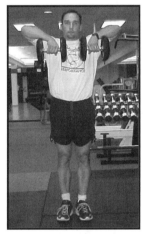

FINISH

DIFFICULTY -	H	H	H
♂ STARTING WEIGHT - 20			
♀ STARTING WEIGHT - 10			

SIDE SHOULDER EXERCISES 197

ALTERNATE DUMBBELL UPRIGHT ROW

MAJOR MUSCLES IN USE:
Medial Deltoid, Trapezius, Upper Portion of Pectoralis Major

STARTING POSITION:
- Stand with feet about shoulder width apart and grasp each dumbbell with an overhand grip. Place your hands so that your palms are facing your legs and the dumbbells and are about 6 – 8 inches apart.
- Allow your arms to straighten so that the dumbbells hang just above your mid- thigh.
- Bend your knees slightly and straighten your back and your shoulders by keeping your chest held high.

EXERCISE MOVEMENT:
- While keeping your chest high, pull one dumbbell up and slightly outwards so that it travels to one side of your body midline.
- Make sure that your elbow always stays above the dumbbell and moves directly out to the side.
- Allow the dumbbell to follow the contour of your body and to stop at the base of your neck or level with you collar bone.
- Lower the dumbbell back to the starting position along the same path that it was raised.
- Repeat the motion with the opposite arm.

EXERCISE TECHNIQUE POINTS:
- Do not allow your elbow to fall below the level of the dumbbell.
- Make sure that you hold your chest high throughout the whole movement.
- Make sure you keep your heels on the floor.
- Do not rock your torso back and forth in order to complete the necessary repetitions.

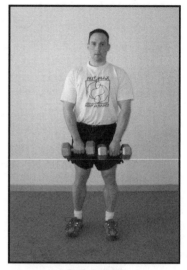
START

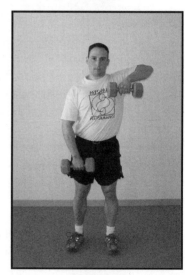
FINISH

DIFFICULTY -	H H H
♂	STARTING WEIGHT - 20
♀	STARTING WEIGHT - 10

HAMMER DUMBBELL UPRIGHT ROW

MAJOR MUSCLES IN USE:
Medial Deltoid, Trapezius, Upper Portion of Pectoralis Major

STARTING POSITION:
- Standing with feet about shoulder width apart, grasp each dumbbell with an overhand grip. Your hands should be positioned on either side of your thighs with your palms facing inwards.
- Allow your arms to straighten so that the dumbbells hang just above the level of your mid-thigh.
- Bend your knees slightly and straighten your back and shoulders by holding your chest high.

EXERCISE MOVEMENT:
- While keeping your chest high, begin by lifting the dumbbells up (following the sides of your torso) towards your shoulders.
- Continue to pull the dumbbells up along the side of your body until you can not lift them any higher.
- Lower the dumbbells back to the starting position along the same path.

EXERCISE TECHNIQUE POINTS:
- Make sure that your chest is held high throughout the whole movement.
- Make sure you keep the heels on the floor.
- Do not rock your torso back and forth in order to complete the necessary repetitions.

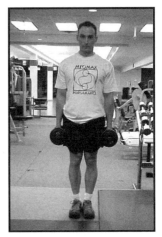

START

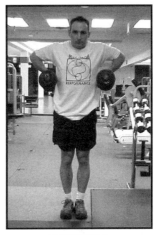

FINISH

DIFFICULTY -	H H H	
♂	STARTING WEIGHT - 20	
♀	STARTING WEIGHT - 12	

SIDE SHOULDER EXERCISES 199

SEATED UPRIGHT ROW

MAJOR MUSCLES IN USE:
Medial Deltoid, Trapezius, Upper Portion of Pectoralis Major

STARTING POSITION:
- Sit on the end of a bench and rest the bar across your thighs. Take an overhand grip on the bar so that your hands are placed about 6 – 8 inches apart.
- Your elbows should be bent and positioned out to your sides.
- Straighten your back and your shoulders by holding your chest high.

EXERCISE MOVEMENT:
- While keeping your chest held high, pull the bar up towards your collarbone.
- Make sure that your elbows always stay above the bar and move directly out to the sides.
- Allow the bar to follow the contour of your body and to stop at the base of your neck or when level with your collarbone.
- Lower the bar back to your thighs along the same path that it was raised.

EXERCISE TECHNIQUE POINTS:
- Do not allow your elbows to fall below the level of the bar.
- Make sure that you keep your chest up throughout the whole movement.
- Do not rock your torso back and forth in order to complete the necessary repetitions.

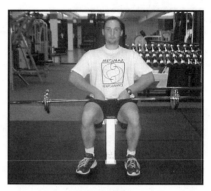
START

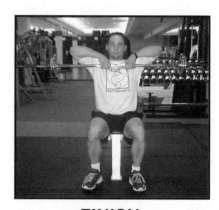
FINISH

DIFFICULTY -	H
♂ STARTING WEIGHT - 50	
♀ STARTING WEIGHT - 25	

SEATED DUMBBELL UPRIGHT ROW

MAJOR MUSCLES IN USE:
Medial Deltoid, Trapezius, Upper Portion of Pectoralis Major

STARTING POSITION:
- Sit on a bench, grasp each dumbbell with an overhand grip and place them at your sides so that the palms of your hands face in towards your body.
- Allow your arms to straighten so that the dumbbells hang below your thighs.
- Straighten your back and your shoulders by keeping your chest held high.

EXERCISE MOVEMENT:
- While keeping your chest high, pull the dumbbells up towards your collarbone so that the dumbbells follow the path of a narrow "A".
- As your hands rise above your thighs and move to the front of your body, twist your palms so that they face your torso.
- Make sure that your elbows always stay above the dumbbells and move directly out to your sides.
- Allow the dumbbells to follow the contour of your body and stop at the base of your neck or at collarbone level.
- Lower the dumbbells back to the starting position along the same path that they were raised.

EXERCISE TECHNIQUE POINTS:
- Do not allow your elbows to fall below the level of the dumbbells.
- Make sure that you keep your chest held high throughout the whole movement.
- Do not rock your torso back and forth in order to complete the necessary repetitions.

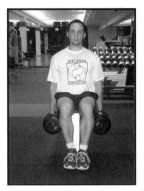

START

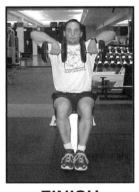

FINISH

DIFFICULTY -	H	H
♂ STARTING WEIGHT - 20		
♀ STARTING WEIGHT - 10		

REAR SHOULDER EXERCISES

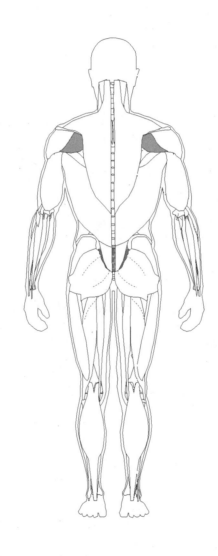

SEATED BENT OVER LATERALS

MAJOR MUSCLES IN USE:
Posterior Deltoid, Middle and Lower Portion of the Trapezius

STARTING POSITION:
- Sit on the end of a flat bench with your feet together and approximately 2 – 3 feet away from the end of the bench.
- Holding a dumbbell in each hand, bend over at the waist so that your chest either touches or comes very close to your thighs.
- Keeping your elbows slightly bent, place the dumbbells behind your feet with your palms facing each other.

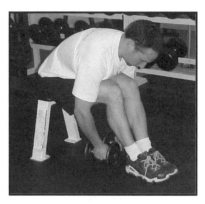

START

EXERCISE MOVEMENT:
- While keeping your elbows slightly bent, begin by lifting the dumbbells up and outwards away from your torso in a semicircular arc. Your arms should travel on a path that is perpendicular to your torso.
- At the end point in the movement, the bar on the dumbbell should be about level with your shoulders and the dumbbells opposite your ears. Your elbows should be still slightly bent.
- As you raise the dumbbells, your palms should always be facing the floor.
- Finish the exercise by returning the dumbbells to the starting position following the same semicircular motion used in raising them.

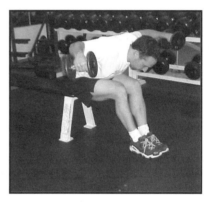

FINISH

EXERCISE TECHNIQUE POINTS:
- Do not bounce your arms off your thighs in order to complete the necessary repetitions.
- Do not allow your elbows to either straighten or bend more than 10°.
- A slight twist of the dumbbells at the top of the motion so that your index finger is lower than your little finger will keep the posterior deltoid in a strong contraction position.
- Do not allow your index finger to rise higher than your little finger.

DIFFICULTY -	H	H	H
♂ STARTING WEIGHT - 10			
♀ STARTING WEIGHT - 5			

BENT OVER LATERALS

MAJOR MUSCLES IN USE:
Posterior Deltoid, Middle and Lower Portion of the Trapezius

STARTING POSITION:
- Stand with your feet about shoulder-width apart and a dumbbell in each hand. Bend over at the waist so that your torso is approximately parallel to the ground.
- Make sure to keep your back flat by bending at the knees and keeping your chest pushed out.
- With your elbows slightly bent, place the dumbbells in front of your legs with your palms facing each other.

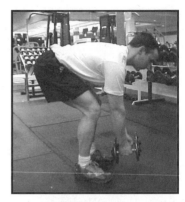

START

EXERCISE MOVEMENT:
- While keeping your elbows slightly bent, begin by lifting the dumbbells up and outwards away from your torso in a semicircular arc. Your arms should travel along a line that is perpendicular to your torso.
- At the end point in the movement the bar on the dumbbell should be about level with your shoulders, the dumbbells directly opposite your ears, and your elbows still slightly bent.
- As you raise the dumbbells, your palms should always face the floor.
- Finish the exercise by returning the dumbbells to the starting position using the same semicircular motion as when they were raised.

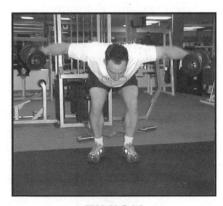

FINISH

EXERCISE TECHNIQUE POINTS:
- Do not round your back by allowing your chest to drop.
- Do not allow your elbows to either straighten or bend more than 10°.
- Slightly twist the dumbbells at the top of the motion so that your index finger is lower than your little finger as this will keep the posterior deltoid in a strong contraction position.
- Do not allow your index finger to rise higher than your little finger.

DIFFICULTY -	⊢ ⊢ ⊢
♂ STARTING WEIGHT - 10	
♀ STARTING WEIGHT - 5	

ONE ARM BENT OVER LATERALS

MAJOR MUSCLES IN USE:
Posterior Deltoid, Middle and Lower Portion of the Trapezius

STARTING POSITION:
- Position yourself on a bench so that one knee and one hand (on the same side of the body) are supporting your body on the bench. The other foot should be placed on the floor with the other hand grasping a dumbbell.
- Allow the dumbbell to hang directly below your shoulder while holding your arm straight. Your back should be flat and shoulders parallel to the floor.

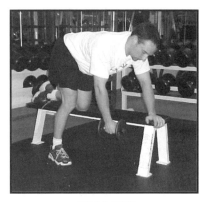

START

EXERCISE MOVEMENT:
- While keeping your elbow slightly bent, begin by lifting the dumbbell up and outwards away from your torso in a semicircular arc. Your arm should travel along a line that is perpendicular to your torso.
- At the end point of the movement, the bar on the dumbbell should be about level with your shoulder and opposite your ear with your elbow still slightly bent.
- As you raise the dumbbell, your palm should always be facing the floor.
- Finish the exercise by returning the dumbbell to the starting position along the same semicircular path that it was raised.

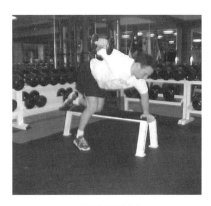

FINISH

EXERCISE TECHNIQUE POINTS:
- Do not round your back by allowing your chest to drop.
- Do not allow your elbow to either straighten or bend more than 10°.
- A slight twist of the dumbbell at the top of the motion (so that your index finger is lower than your little finger) will keep the posterior deltoid muscle in a strong contraction position.

DIFFICULTY -	⊢⊣ ⊢⊣ ⊢⊣	
♂	STARTING WEIGHT - 10	
♀	STARTING WEIGHT - 5	

REAR DELT KICKBACKS

MAJOR MUSCLES IN USE:
Posterior Deltoid, Middle and Lower Portion of the Trapezius

STARTING POSITION:
- Position yourself on a bench so that one knee and one hand on the same side of the body are supporting your torso on the bench. The other foot should be placed on the floor and the other hand grasping a dumbbell.
- Allow the dumbbell to hang directly below your shoulder with your arm in a slightly bent position and your palm facing in towards your body.
- Your back should be flat and shoulders parallel with the floor.

EXERCISE MOVEMENT:
- While keeping your elbow in a slightly bent position, start by moving the dumbbell back along the side of your body in an upwards arc by only allowing movement at your shoulder joint.
- Your arm should swing alongside your body like a pendulum while your hand twists upwards.
- At the end point in the movement your hand should be level with your hip and your palm facing upwards.
- Finish the exercise by returning the dumbbell to the starting position along the same path that it was raised.

EXERCISE TECHNIQUE POINTS:
- Do not round your back by allowing your chest to drop.
- Do not allow your elbow to bend.
- If you feel the exercise too much in the back of your arm (triceps muscle), try bending the elbow a bit more.

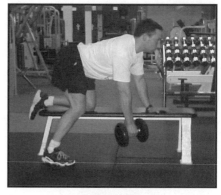

START

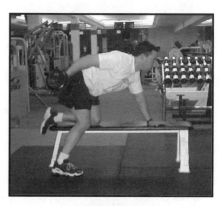

FINISH

DIFFICULTY -	H H H H
♂ STARTING WEIGHT - 12	
♀ STARTING WEIGHT - 8	

HIGH PULLBACKS

MAJOR MUSCLES IN USE:
Posterior Deltoid, Middle and Lower Portion of the Trapezius

STARTING POSITION:
- Using the close grip handle, sit at the pulldown machine and take an overhand grip with your palms facing each other.
- Begin with arms straight and your chest up, leaning as far back as necessary so that your arms form a 90° angle with your body.

EXERCISE MOVEMENT:
- While keeping your elbows high and pointing directly out, arch your back by raising your chest and pull the bar down close to your upper chest.
- Return the bar to the starting position at a moderate pace. When finished, your arms should once again be straight.

EXERCISE TECHNIQUE POINTS:
- Do not round your back by allowing your chest to lower while you pull down.
- Do not rock back and forth in order to complete the repetitions.
- Always make sure your arms and elbows are pointing straight out to the sides and are away from your body.

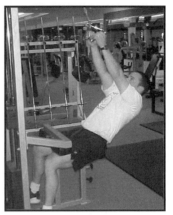

START

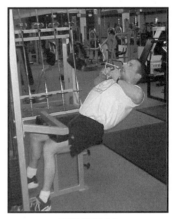

FINISH

DIFFICULTY -	⊢ ⊢ ⊢
♂ STARTING WEIGHT - 60	
♀ STARTING WEIGHT - 30	

REAR SHOULDER EXERCISES 207

DUMBBELL HIGH PULLBACKS

MAJOR MUSCLES IN USE:
Posterior Deltoid, Middle and Lower Portion of the Trapezius

STARTING POSITION:
- Stand with feet about shoulder width apart and your knees slightly bent.
- Bend over at the waist with your hips and buttocks pushed out forming a slight curve in your lower back. Your upper back should be flat. Your upper back will flatten if you keep your chest up.
- Grasp two dumbbells and position your hands so that your palms are facing back towards your feet while keeping your arms are straight. Your abdominal muscles should be tensed. Your upper back should be just parallel to the floor.

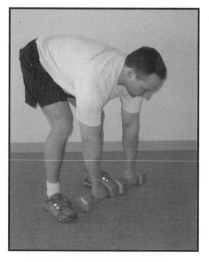

START

EXERCISE MOVEMENT:
- While keeping your upper body stationary and your back flat, pull the dumbbells up and out towards the sides of your shoulders. Make sure you try and keep your elbows pointing out away from your body.
- Pull the dumbbells up and out as high as you can so that your upper arm is at least parallel to the floor and perpendicular to your body. Reverse the motion by lowering the dumbbells down and inwards so that the dumbbells return to the starting position.

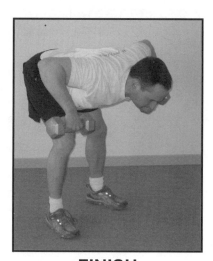

FINISH

EXERCISE TECHNIQUE POINTS:
- Keep your chest and buttocks pushed out so that you have a slight arch in your lower back while your upper back remains flat.
- Do not allow your upper body to rise as if you were beginning to stand up.
- You may wish to wear a belt on this exercise to help support the trunk.
- Squeeze your shoulder blades together at the top portion of the movement to activate the middle portion of your trapezius.

DIFFICULTY -	H H H
♂ STARTING WEIGHT - 15	
♀ STARTING LEVEL - 8	

BENCH PULLBACKS

MAJOR MUSCLES IN USE:
Posterior Deltoid, Middle and Lower Portion of the Trapezius

STARTING POSITION:
- Position yourself on a high bench (either a specially designed adjustable bench or a normal bench on blocks) so that you are lying on your stomach with your arms hanging down on either side. Your fingers should not touch the floor.
- In each hand grasp a dumbbell and allow the dumbbells to hang directly below your shoulders when your arms are straight with your palms facing back towards your feet.

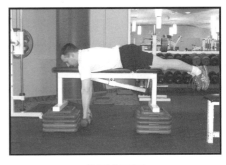

START

EXERCISE MOVEMENT:
- While keeping your elbows pointing out away from your body, pull the dumbbells up with both arms towards the sides of your shoulders.
- Pull the dumbbells up and out as high as you can so that your upper arm is at least parallel to the floor and perpendicular to your body. Reverse the motion by lowering the dumbbells down and inwards so that the dumbbells return to the starting position.

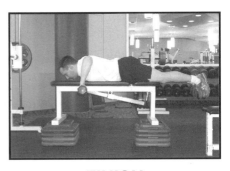

FINISH

EXERCISE TECHNIQUE POINTS:
- Do not round your upper back. Make sure it stays parallel with the bench while maintaining a slight arch in your lower back.
- Do not allow yourself to twist or arch your upper body so that your chest rises off the bench when performing your repetitions.
- Squeeze your shoulder blades together at the top portion of the movement to activate the middle portion of your trapezius.

DIFFICULTY -	⊢⊢	
♂	STARTING WEIGHT - 15	
♀	STARTING LEVEL - 8	

SEATED HIGH PULLBACKS

MAJOR MUSCLES IN USE:
Posterior Deltoid, Middle and Lower Portion of the Trapezius

STARTING POSITION:
- Sitting in front of a low pulley, place your feet on either side of the cable about 6 inches in front of the pulley. Many commercial gyms have a specialised machine to do this specific movement. Grasp a long bar handle with your hands placed a bit wider apart than shoulder width. Sit up straight with your chest high and your knees bent. Your torso should stay in this position throughout the exercise.

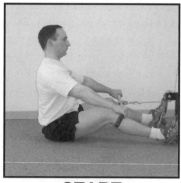

START

EXERCISE MOVEMENT:
- While keeping your torso stationary and your abdominal muscles tensed, pull the bar towards your mid-chest. Make sure your elbows always point outwards as you pull the bar back.
- Pull the handle in until it lightly touches your chest. Reverse the motion so that the handle returns to the same place as when you began your repetition.

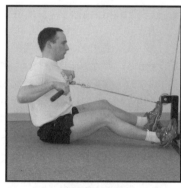

FINISH

EXERCISE TECHNIQUE POINTS:
- Straighten your back by keeping your chest high so that you have a slight arch in your lower back.
- Do not allow yourself to sway excessively when performing your repetitions. A very slight swaying of the torso is acceptable. However, too much may indicate you are using a weight that is too heavy.
- Squeeze your shoulder blades together at the top portion of the movement to activate the middle portion of your trapezius.
- Do not allow your wrists to bend near the end of the motion.

DIFFICULTY -	H H	
♂	STARTING WEIGHT - 60	
♀	STARTING LEVEL - 30	

CABLE BENT OVER LATERALS

MAJOR MUSCLES IN USE:
Posterior Deltoid, Middle and Lower Portion of the Trapezius

STARTING POSITION:
- Position yourself in the middle of a cable crossover machine or between two low pulleys with a single handle attached to each of the cables.
- Stand with feet about shoulder width apart and grab the handles from each low pulley so that they are in opposite hands. Bend over at the waist so that your torso is approximately parallel to the ground.
- Make sure to keep your back flat by bending at the knees and keeping your chest pushed out.
- With you elbows slightly bent, position the handles in front of your legs with your palms facing each other.

EXERCISE MOVEMENT:
- While keeping your elbows slightly bent, begin by lifting the handles outwards away from your torso in an arc. Your arms should travel along a line perpendicular to your torso and the cables should cross in the middle.
- At the end point in the movement, the handles should be about level with your shoulders and opposite your ears.
- As you raise the handles, your palms should always be facing the floor.
- Finish the exercise by returning the handles to the starting position back along the same path followed in raising them.

EXERCISE TECHNIQUE POINTS:
- Do not round your back by allowing your chest to drop.
- Do not allow your elbows to either straighten or bend more than 10°.
- Do not allow your index finger to rise higher than your little finger.

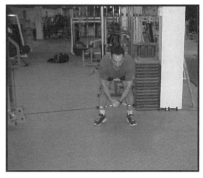

START

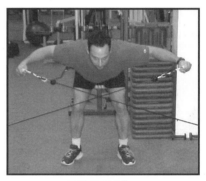

FINISH

DIFFICULTY -	H	H	H
♂ STARTING WEIGHT - 10			
♀ STARTING WEIGHT - 5			

ONE ARM CABLE REAR LATERALS

MAJOR MUSCLES IN USE:
Posterior Deltoid, Middle and Lower Portion of the Trapezius

STARTING POSITION:
- Position yourself with feet shoulder width apart beside a low pulley and bend over at the waist so that your back is approximately parallel to the floor.
- The hand closest to the pulley should support your body by pushing on your thigh while the other hand grasps the single handle attached to the cable.
- Position the handle so that it is at the mid-line of your torso.
- Your back should be flat and shoulders square with the floor.

EXERCISE MOVEMENT:
- While keeping your elbow slightly bent, begin by lifting the handle outwards and directly to the side of your torso in along a semicircular arc.
- At the end point in the movement, the bar on the handle should be about level with your shoulders and opposite your ears.
- As you raise the handle, your palm should always be facing the floor. Keeping your elbow slightly bent.
- Finish the exercise by returning the handle to the starting position back along the same path as when you raised it.

EXERCISE TECHNIQUE POINTS:
- Do not round your back by allowing your chest to drop.
- Do not allow your elbow to either straighten or bend more than 10°.
- A slight twist of the handle at the top of the motion (so that your index finger is lower than your little finger) will keep the posterior deltoid muscle in a strong contraction position.
- Do not allow your index finger to rise higher than your little finger.

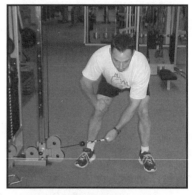

START

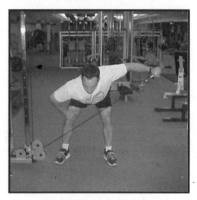

FINISH

DIFFICULTY -	H	H	H
♂ STARTING WEIGHT - 10			
♀ STARTING WEIGHT - 5			

INCLINE BENCH REAR LATERALS

MAJOR MUSCLES IN USE:
Posterior Deltoid, Middle and Lower Portion of the Trapezius

STARTING POSITION:
- Position yourself by lying on your stomach, face down, on an inclining bench set at about 40°. Your chest should rest against the backrest and your legs should be placed off and to either side of the bench.
- Take a dumbbell in each hand and let your arms hang down on either side of the bench. Either turn your head to one side or position your upper body higher on the back rest so that your head is above the top portion of the bench.
- Bend your elbows slightly and position your palms facing each other.

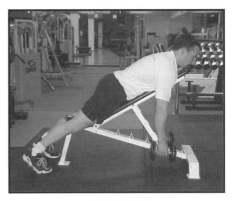

START

EXERCISE MOVEMENT:
- While keeping your elbows slightly bent, begin by lifting the dumbbells outwards and away from the starting position. Your arms should travel along a line perpendicular to your torso.
- At the end point in the movement, the bars on the dumbbells should be about level with your shoulders and opposite your ears. Your elbows should be still slightly bent.
- Your palms should always be facing the floor as you raise the dumbbells.
- Finish the exercise by returning the dumbbells to the starting position along the same path used in raising them.

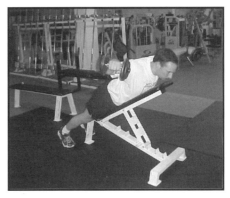

FINISH

EXERCISE TECHNIQUE POINTS:
- Do not allow your elbows to either straighten or bend more than 10°.
- A slight twist of the dumbbells at the top of the motion (so that your index finger is lower than your little finger) will keep the posterior deltoid muscle in a strong contraction position.
- Do not allow your index finger to rise higher than your little finger.

DIFFICULTY -	⊢ ⊢ ⊢	
♂	STARTING WEIGHT - 10	
♀	STARTING WEIGHT - 5	

REAR SHOULDER EXERCISES 213

STANDING ONE ARM CABLE REAR LATERALS

MAJOR MUSCLES IN USE:
Posterior Deltoid, Middle and Lower Portion of the Trapezius

STARTING POSITION:
- Stand beside the pulldown machine at a distance of a little more than arms-length away.
- Grasp the single handle from the high pulley with the hand that is farthest away from the machine. Place your feet shoulder-width apart and grab on to the pulldown machine with your free hand.
- Your arm should be slightly bent and positioned in front of your body so that the handle is at your body's midline.

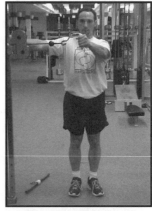

START

EXERCISE MOVEMENT:
- While keeping your elbow locked at a slightly bent angle and your hand always vertical, begin the exercise by bringing the handle out and away from your body. Your hand should move along a semicircular path that is slightly more than parallel to the floor.
- At the end point in the movement, the handle should be about level with your chin and as far back as possible. You should raise your chest by arching your upper back in order to hold the proper exercise form.
- Remember to keep your elbow slightly bent. Your arm should stay roughly parallel to the floor.
- Finish the exercise by returning the handle back to the starting position along the same path that it was raised.

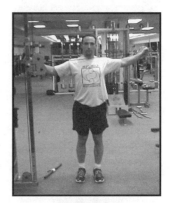

FINISH

EXERCISE TECHNIQUE POINTS:
- Remember to stand upright with your back straight.
- Do not allow your elbow to either straighten or bend more than 10°.
- Do not twist the handle during any part of the movement.

DIFFICULTY - H H H		
♂	STARTING WEIGHT - 15	
♀	STARTING WEIGHT - 10	

REAR CABLE CROSS-OVER

MAJOR MUSCLES IN USE:
Posterior Deltoid, Latissimus Dorsi, Teres Major

STARTING POSITION:
- This exercise requires a special cable crossover machine or an exercise set-up of two pulldown machines facing each other.
- Grasp each single handle from the high pulleys with each hand and position yourself in the middle of the machine. Place your feet shoulder width apart and position your hands directly above your head.
- Your arms should be slightly bent and your elbows should be positioned outwards and directed towards the high pulleys.

EXERCISE MOVEMENT:
- While keeping your elbows slightly bent, begin by bringing the handles outwards and down towards the floor. Your hands should move together along a semicircular path.
- At the end point in the movement, the handles should be about level with your shoulders and your elbows slightly bent. Your chest should also be slightly raised by arching your back upwards.
- Finish the exercise by returning the handles back to the starting position following the same semicircular motion used in lowering them.

EXERCISE TECHNIQUE POINTS:
- Remember to keep your elbows slightly bent and your palms facing upwards at the bottom portion of the movement.
- Do not twist the handles during any part of the movement.

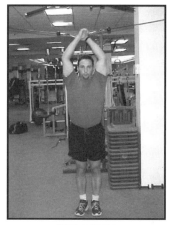

START

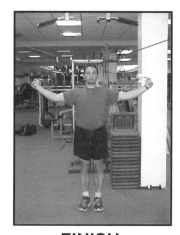

FINISH

DIFFICULTY -	⊢ ⊢ ⊢	
♂	STARTING WEIGHT - 15	
♀	STARTING WEIGHT - 10	

REAR SHOULDER EXERCISES 215

ROTATOR CUFF EXERCISES

The Rotator Cuff Muscles
are a group of several
different muscles that help
stabilize the shoulder joint
and are covered by the
shoulder muscles

LYING EXTERNAL ROTATION

MAJOR MUSCLES IN USE:
Rotator Cuff Muscles

STARTING POSITION:
- Lie on your side on top of a flat bench.
- The arm holding the dumbbell should be bent at 90° so that your upper arm rests on your upper side and your forearm crosses in front of your midsection.

EXERCISE MOVEMENT:
- While keeping your upper arm pressed into your torso and your elbow stationary, begin by rotating your upper arm so that the dumbbell rises along a semicircular path away from your body.
- Only the forearm and upper arm should move while the elbow remains at the same position on your side.
- Finish with the dumbbell as high as possible and your arm rotated away from your body.
- Return the weight back to the starting position while not allowing your elbow or upper arm to slide forwards or backwards.

EXERCISE TECHNIQUE POINTS:
- Do not allow the dumbbell to lower so fast that you cannot control it.
- Do not allow your body to roll to one side in order to complete the repetitions.
- Do not allow your elbow to move or your upper arm to rise off your torso.

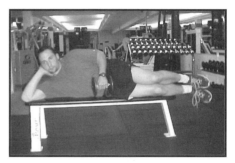

START

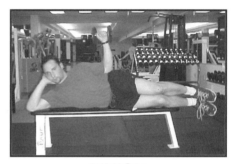

FINISH

DIFFICULTY -	⊢⊣	⊢⊣
♂ STARTING WEIGHT - 10		
♀ STARTING WEIGHT - 5		

ROTATOR CUFF EXERCISES

EXTERNAL ROTATION

MAJOR MUSCLES IN USE:
Rotator Cuff Muscles

STARTING POSITION:
- Sit beside a bench and place your upper arm and forearm on the bench.
- The arm holding the dumbbell should be bent at 90° and should be as flat as possible against the bench.

EXERCISE MOVEMENT:
- While keeping your arm at 90° and your upper arm in contact with the bench, rotate your arm so that your forearm and the hand holding the dumbbell rises along an arcing path.
- The elbow must remain at the same position on the bench.
- Finish with the dumbbell held as high as possible and your arm rotated so that your forearm is perpendicular to the floor.
- Return the weight to the starting position while not allowing your elbow to rise off the bench.

EXERCISE TECHNIQUE POINTS:
- Do not allow the dumbbell to lower so fast that you can not control it.
- Do not allow your elbow to slide back and forth or your upper arm to rise off the bench.

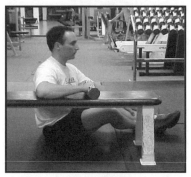

START

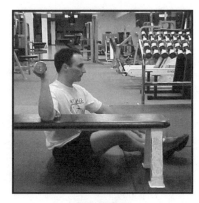

FINISH

DIFFICULTY -	H	H
♂ STARTING WEIGHT - 10		
♀ STARTING WEIGHT - 5		

ROTATOR CUFF EXERCISES 218

CABLE EXTERNAL ROTATION

MAJOR MUSCLES IN USE:
Rotator Cuff Muscles

STARTING POSITION:
- Position yourself facing the front of an overhead pulley machine. Grasp the single handle with one hand and take several steps back away from the machine so that there is tension on the cable.
- Position your upper arm parallel to the floor with your elbow in line with your shoulders. Your forearm should also be parallel to the floor but with your elbow bent at 90°. Grasp a single handle with your palm forward while your non-exercising hand rests on your hip or abdomen.
- Tense your abdominal and lower back muscles to stabilize your torso.

EXERCISE MOVEMENT:
- While keeping your upper arm stationary, rotate your arm upwards and away from the machine moving in a semicircular motion so that only the forearm moves while the elbow remains in the same position.
- Finish with your arm fully rotated upwards and back so that your hand is either directly above or slightly behind your elbow.
- Return the weight to the starting position while not allowing your elbow to move.

EXERCISE TECHNIQUE POINTS:
- Do not allow your elbow to move as you raise and lower the weight back to the starting position.
- Do not bend your wrist in order to complete the repetitions
- Keep your abdominal muscles tensed and one leg forward in order to help keep your balance and proper form.

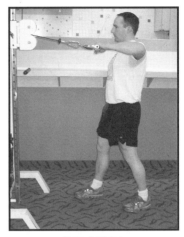

START

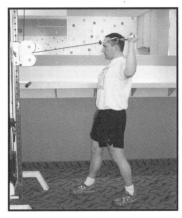

FINISH

DIFFICULTY -	H	H	H
♂ STARTING WEIGHT - 15			
♀ STARTING WEIGHT - 10			

ROTATOR CUFF EXERCISES 219

LATERAL EXTERNAL ROTATION

MAJOR MUSCLES IN USE:
 Rotator Cuff Muscles

STARTING POSITION:
- Stand with your feet shoulder width apart with your shoulders even with your hips and your chest held high.
- Grasp a dumbbell with each hand and position your upper arms parallel to the floor with your elbows in line with your shoulders. Your forearms should also be parallel to the floor with your elbows bent at 90°.
- Tense your abdominal and lower back muscles to stabilize your torso.

EXERCISE MOVEMENT:
- While keeping your upper arms stationary, rotate your forearms upwards and back in a semicircular motion so that only the forearms move while the elbows remain in the same position.
- Finish with your arms fully rotated upwards and back so that your hands are either directly above or slightly behind your elbows.
- Return the weight to the starting position while not allowing your elbows to move.

EXERCISE TECHNIQUE POINTS:
- Do not allow your elbows to move as you raise and lower the weights back to the starting position.
- Do not bend your wrists in order to complete the repetitions.
- Keep your abdominal muscles tensed in order to help keep your balance and proper form.
- You may also perform the exercise one arm at a time.

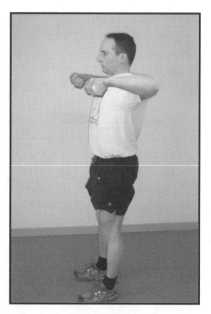

START

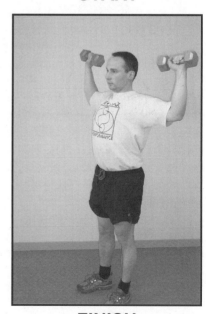

FINISH

DIFFICULTY -	⊢⊢ ⊢⊢ ⊢⊢
♂ STARTING WEIGHT - 10	
♀ STARTING WEIGHT - 5	

ROTATOR CUFF EXERCISES

CROSS BODY CABLE EXTERNAL ROTATION

MAJOR MUSCLES IN USE:
Rotator Cuff Muscles

STARTING POSITION:
- Stand in front of an adjustable pulley positioned at the level of your elbow with feet about shoulder width apart. Your body should be positioned perpendicular to the machine so that one side of your body is close to the pulley.
- Grasp a single handle attached to the cable and position your arm so that your upper arm and elbow are touching your side and your elbow is bent at 90°.
- Your forearm should be positioned across your abdominal region with your hand still at the same level of your elbow.

EXERCISE MOVEMENT:
- While keeping your upper arm stationary, rotate your arm outwards across your body moving along a semicircular path so that only the forearm moves while the elbow remains in the same position.
- Finish with your forearm fully rotated outwards as far as possible with your hand still at the same level of your elbow.
- Return the weight to the starting position by reversing the motion that it was lifted.

EXERCISE TECHNIQUE POINTS:
- Do not allow your elbow to move away from your body as you raise and lower the weight.
- Do not bend your wrist in order to complete the repetitions.
- Make sure your elbow stays bent at a 90° angle at all times.
- Keep your abdominal muscles tensed and one leg forward in order to help keep your balance and proper form.

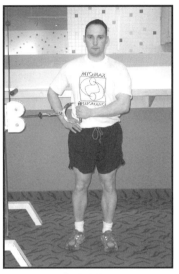

START

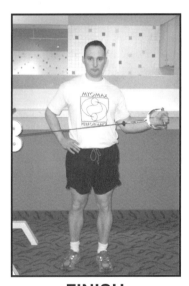

FINISH

DIFFICULTY -	H H H	
♂	STARTING WEIGHT - 10	
♀	STARTING WEIGHT - 5	

ROTATOR CUFF EXERCISES 221

CROSS BODY CABLE INTERNAL ROTATION

MAJOR MUSCLES IN USE:
Rotator Cuff Muscles

STARTING POSITION:
- Stand in front of an adjustable pulley positioned at the level of your elbow with feet about shoulder width apart. Your body should be positioned perpendicular to the machine so that one side of your body is close to the pulley.
- Grasp a single handle attached to the cable and position your arm so that your upper arm and elbow are touching your side and your elbow is bent at 90°.
- Depending on your shoulder flexibility, your hand should be placed directly in front of your elbow or slightly to the outside.

EXERCISE MOVEMENT:
- While keeping your upper arm stationary, rotate your arm inwards across your body moving in a semicircular motion so that only the forearm moves while the elbow remains in the same position.
- Finish with your forearm across your abdominal region fully rotated inwards with your hand still at the same level of your elbow.
- Return the weight to the starting position by reversing the motion that it was lifted.

EXERCISE TECHNIQUE POINTS:
- Do not allow your elbow to move away from your body as you raise and lower the weight.
- Do not bend your wrist in order to complete the repetitions.
- Make sure your elbow stays bent at a 90° angle at all times.
- Keep your abdominal muscles tensed and one leg forward in order to help keep your balance and proper form.

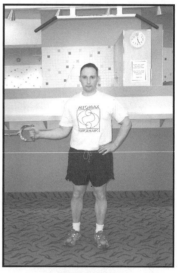

START

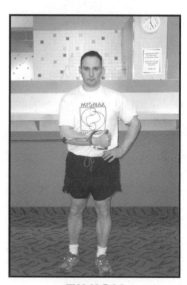

FINISH

DIFFICULTY -	H	H	H
♂ STARTING WEIGHT - 20			
♀ STARTING WEIGHT - 10			

CABLE INTERNAL ROTATION

MAJOR MUSCLES IN USE:
Rotator Cuff Muscles

STARTING POSITION:
- Position yourself with your back facing the front of an overhead pulley machine. Grasp the single handle with one hand and take several steps forward away from the machine so that there is tension on the cable.
- Position your upper arm parallel to the floor with your elbow in line with your shoulders. Your forearm should be vertical with your elbow bent at 90°. Grasp a single handle with your palm facing forward while your non-exercising hand rests on your hip or abdomen.
- Tense your abdominal and lower back muscles to stabilize your torso.

EXERCISE MOVEMENT:
- While keeping your upper arm stationary, rotate your arm downwards and forwards away from the machine. Your hand should move along a semicircular path so that only the forearm moves while the elbow remains in the same position.
- Finish with your arm fully rotated forwards so that your hand is directly in front of or slightly below the level of your elbow.
- Return the weight to the starting position while not allowing your elbow to move.

EXERCISE TECHNIQUE POINTS:
- Do not allow your elbow to move as you raise and lower the weight.
- Do not bend your wrist in order to complete the repetitions.
- Keep your abdominal muscles tensed and one leg forward in order to help keep your balance and proper form.

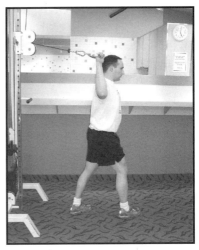

START

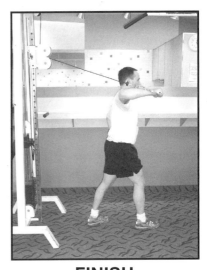

FINISH

DIFFICULTY -	⊢ ⊢ ⊢	
♂	STARTING WEIGHT - 10	
♀	STARTING WEIGHT - 5	

ROTATOR CUFF EXERCISES   223

INTERNAL SIDE ROTATION

MAJOR MUSCLES IN USE:
Rotator Cuff Muscles

STARTING POSITION:
- Lie on your side on top of a flat bench. Grasp a dumbbell in your lower hand.
- The arm holding the dumbbell should be bent at 90° and in front of your body.
- Your upper arm should rest on the bench and press against the front of your torso while your forearm hangs over the bench parallel to the floor but perpendicular to your torso.

EXERCISE MOVEMENT:
- While keeping your upper arm and your elbow stationary, begin by rotating your arm at the shoulder inwards so that the dumbbell rises along an arcing path crossing your torso.
- Only the forearm should move and the upper arm to rotate while the elbow remains in the same position.
- Finish with the dumbbell raised as high as possible and your arm rotated inwards towards your chest.
- Return the weight to the starting position while not allowing your elbow to move forwards or backwards.

EXERCISE TECHNIQUE POINTS:
- Do not allow the dumbbell to lower so fast that you cannot control it.
- Do not allow your body to roll to one side in order to complete the repetitions.
- Do not allow the elbow of your exercising arm to move back and forth during the exercise.

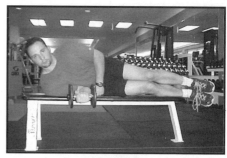

START

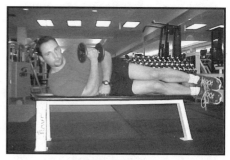

FINISH

DIFFICULTY -	H	H	
♂	STARTING WEIGHT - 15		
♀	STARTING WEIGHT - 8		

ROTATOR CUFF EXERCISES

LYING INTERNAL ROTATION

MAJOR MUSCLES IN USE:
Rotator Cuff Muscles

STARTING POSITION:
- Lie on your back on the floor and hold a dumbbell in one hand.
- The arm holding the dumbbell should be bent upwards at 90° at the elbow so that your forearm is perpendicular to the floor. Your upper arm should be placed at a 90° angle to your torso.

EXERCISE MOVEMENT:
- While keeping your elbow stationary, begin by rotating your upper arm at the shoulder backwards so that the dumbbell lowers in a semicircular arc towards the floor.
- Only the forearm should move while the elbow and upper arm remains in contact with the floor.
- Finish with the dumbbell as low as possible so that your forearm is touching or is very close to the floor.
- Return the weight to the starting position while not allowing your elbow to move forwards or backwards.

EXERCISE TECHNIQUE POINTS:
- Do not allow the dumbbell to lower so fast that you cannot control it.
- Do not allow your elbow to move forwards, backwards, or rise off the floor.

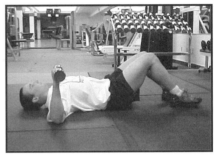

START

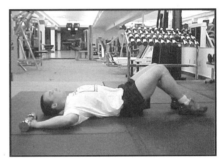

FINISH

DIFFICULTY - ⊢⊣ ⊢⊣	
♂	STARTING WEIGHT - 15
♀	STARTING WEIGHT - 8

TRICEPS EXERCISES

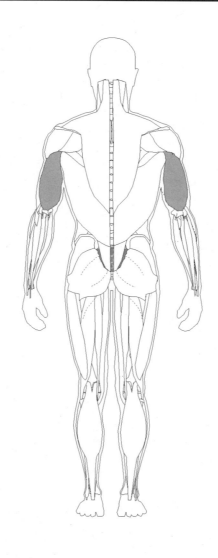

TRICEPS PUSHDOWNS

MAJOR MUSCLES IN USE:
Triceps Brachii

STARTING POSITION:
- Standing with knees slightly bent in front of an overhead pulley machine, take an overhand grip on the bar, or rope handle, with hands about shoulder width apart.
- Begin with arms bent so that the bar is at mid-chest level.
- Elbows should be tucked into your sides and should not move during the exercise.
- A slight forward lean is allowed and may make the exercise more comfortable.

EXERCISE MOVEMENT:
- While keeping your upper arms stationary, begin by extending the arms so that only the forearms are moving and the elbows remain in the same position.
- At midpoint in the motion your arms should be bent at 90° with your forearms parallel to the floor and your upper arms perpendicular to the floor.
- Finish with arms fully extended so that the whole arm is straight and the bar is at mid-thigh level.
- Return the weight to the starting position while not allowing your elbows to move forward.

EXERCISE TECHNIQUE POINTS:
- Do not lean too far forward.
- Do not allow your elbows to move forward as you bring the weight back up.
- Do not allow the bar to come up higher than mid-chest.

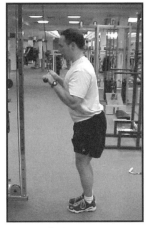

START

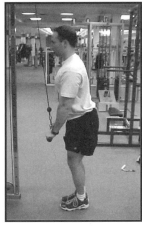

FINISH

DIFFICULTY - ⊢⊣ ⊢⊣		
♂	STARTING WEIGHT - 50	
♀	STARTING WEIGHT - 30	

REVERSE GRIP TRICEPS PUSHDOWNS

MAJOR MUSCLES IN USE:
Triceps Brachii

STARTING POSITION:
- Standing with knees slightly bent in front of an overhead pulley machine, take an underhand grip on the bar with hands about shoulder width apart.
- Begin with arms bent so that the bar is at the level of your mid-chest.
- Elbows should be tucked into your sides and should not move during the exercise.
- A slight forward lean is allowed and may make the exercise more comfortable.

EXERCISE MOVEMENT:
- While keeping your upper arms stationary, begin by extending the arms so that only the forearms are moving and the elbows remain in the same position.
- At midpoint in the motion, your arms should be bent at 90° with your forearms parallel to the floor and your upper arms perpendicular to the floor.
- Finish with the bar at mid-thigh level and arms fully extended so that the whole arm is straight.
- Return the weight to the starting position while not allowing your elbows to move forwards.

EXERCISE TECHNIQUE POINTS:
- Do not lean too far forward.
- Do not allow your elbows to move forward as you bring the weight back up.
- Do not allow the bar to come up higher than mid-chest.
- If you cannot keep a full grip on the bar try placing your hands wider apart.

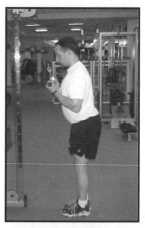

START

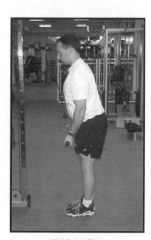

FINISH

DIFFICULTY -	�muⴕⴕ
♂	STARTING WEIGHT - 45
♀	STARTING WEIGHT - 25

HIGH PULLEY TRICEPS EXTENSION

MAJOR MUSCLES IN USE:
Triceps Brachii

STARTING POSITION:
- Position yourself with your back facing the front of an overhead pulley machine. Grasp the rope handle with both hands and lean forward away from the machine by taking a large step forward and inclining your torso forward.
- Begin with your arms fully bent so that your hands are behind your head and your elbows are close to your ears.
- Your torso should be at about a 45° angle to the floor.

EXERCISE MOVEMENT:
- Keeping your upper arms stationary, extend the arms in a semicircular motion so that only the forearms are moving and the elbows remain in the same position.
- Finish with your arms fully extended so that the elbows are locked.
- Return the weight to the starting position while not allowing your elbows to move.

EXERCISE TECHNIQUE POINTS:
- Do not lean too far forward so that the cable hits you in the back of the head.
- Do not allow your elbows to move as you bring the weight back to the start.
- Keep your abdominal muscles tensed and one leg forward in order to help keep your balance and proper form.

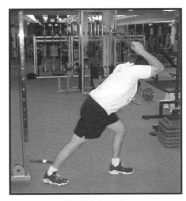

START

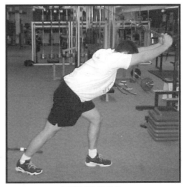

FINISH

DIFFICULTY -	H H H	
♂	STARTING WEIGHT - 50	
♀	STARTING WEIGHT - 25	

ONE ARM HIGH PULLEY TRICEPS EXTENSION

MAJOR MUSCLES IN USE:
Triceps Brachii

STARTING POSITION:
- Position yourself with your back facing the front of an overhead pulley machine. Grasp the single handle with one hand and lean forward, away from the machine.
- Position your hand holding the single handle with your palm forward while your non-exercising hand supports your elbow.
- Begin with your arm fully bent so that your hand is behind your head and your elbow is close to your ears.
- Your torso should be at about a 60° angle to the floor.

EXERCISE MOVEMENT:
- While keeping your upper arm stationary, extend the arm in a semicircular motion so that only the forearm moves while the elbow remains in the same position.
- Finish with your arm fully extended so that the elbow is locked and your wrist is slightly bent back with your palm facing forward.
- Return the weight to the starting position while not allowing your elbow to move.

EXERCISE TECHNIQUE POINTS:
- Do not allow your elbow to move as you bring the weight back to the starting position.
- Keep your abdominal muscles tensed and one leg forward in order to help keep your balance and proper form.

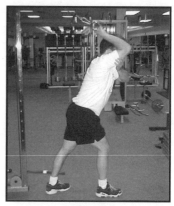
START

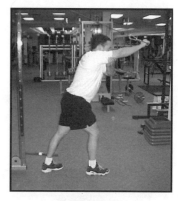
FINISH

DIFFICULTY -	H	H	H
♂ STARTING WEIGHT - 20			
♀ STARTING WEIGHT - 10			

CLOSE GRIP PRESS

MAJOR MUSCLES IN USE:
Triceps Brachii, Anterior Deltoid, Medial Deltoid, Pectoralis Major, Serratus Anterior

STARTING POSITION:
- Lie flat on a bench press bench and position yourself so that your eyes are right below the bar resting on the uprights.
- Use an overhand grip with hands about 12 – 16 inches apart.
- With your feet flat on the floor lift the bar off the uprights and position it right above your shoulders. Your arms should be straight up so that your wrists, elbows, and shoulders are all in line.

EXERCISE MOVEMENT:
- Lower the bar down to the upper portion of your chest following the natural movement pattern of your shoulders.
- Your elbows should be kept close to your sides to allow the triceps muscles to do the majority of the work.
- Let the barbell lightly touch the middle of your upper chest and then push it back up following the same path as when you lowered it.

EXERCISE TECHNIQUE POINTS:
- Do not bounce the barbell off your chest.
- Do not allow your midsection to rise up causing excessive arching in your lower back.
- Your feet should remain on the floor and your hips and upper back should remain on the bench.
- Make sure you do not allow the bar to twist (one side closer to your feet and one side closer to your head) as this could lead to shoulder problems in the future.

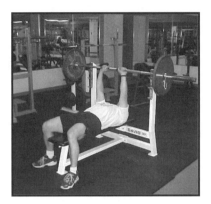

START

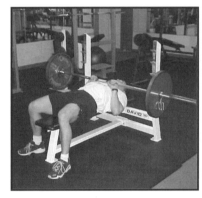

FINISH

DIFFICULTY -	H	
♂	STARTING WEIGHT - 55	
♀	STARTING WEIGHT - 25	

TRICEPS EXERCISES

LYING TRICEPS EXTENSION

MAJOR MUSCLES IN USE:
Triceps Brachii, Serratus Anterior

STARTING POSITION:
- Lying flat on a flat bench, hold an EZ curl bar at arms length directly above your forehead so that your arms are locked and supporting the weight.
- Use a comfortable overhand grip with your hands positioned on the bent portion of the bar. Your hands should be about 6 – 10 inches apart.
- The angle between your arms and the floor should be approximately 70° to the floor.

EXERCISE MOVEMENT:
- While keeping your upper arms stationary, begin by bending at the elbow and lower the bar in a semicircular motion so that only the forearms are moving and the elbows remain locked in the same position.
- Finish with the bar lightly touching the middle of the top of your head while your elbows stay close together.
- Return the weight to the starting position while not allowing your elbows or your upper arms to move.

EXERCISE TECHNIQUE POINTS:
- Do not allow the barbell to lower so fast so that you cannot control it.
- Do not allow your midsection to rise up causing excessive arching in your lower back.
- Your hips and upper back should remain on the bench.
- Do not allow your elbows or your upper arms to move excessively as you lower or raise the weight.

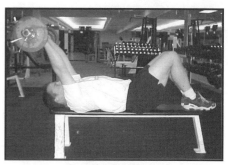

START

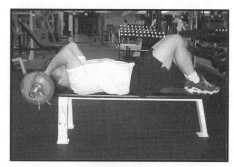

FINISH

DIFFICULTY -	H	H	H
♂ STARTING WEIGHT - 45			
♀ STARTING WEIGHT - 25			

BALL LYING TRICEPS EXTENSION

MAJOR MUSCLES IN USE:
Triceps Brachii, Serratus Anterior

STARTING POSITION:
- Lying on top of an exercise ball, position your body so that your weight is distributed across your shoulders, neck and upper back. Once in position your hips should be held high so that your knees, hips and shoulders are all in a line.
- Position your hands on a dumbbell so that they are both at one end of the dumbbell and are either cupping the bell or are gripping the bar with one hand over top of the other. The dumbbell should be directly above your forehead so that your arms are locked and supporting the weight.
- The angle between your arms and the floor should be approximately 70° to the floor.

EXERCISE MOVEMENT:
- While keeping your upper arm stationary, begin by bending at the elbow and lower the dumbbell in a semicircular motion so that only the forearms are moving and the elbows remain locked in the same position.
- Finish with the bell lightly touching the ball with your elbows staying close together.
- Return the weight to the starting position while not allowing your elbows or your upper arms to move.

EXERCISE TECHNIQUE POINTS:
- Do not allow the dumbbell to lower so fast that you cannot control it.
- Do not allow your midsection to rise up causing excessive arching in your lower back.
- Do not let your hips drop so that they fall out of line with your knees and shoulders.
- Do not allow your elbows or your upper arms to move excessively as you lower or raise the weight.
- To help with balance keep your abdominal and lower back muscles tensed and try taking a wider stance with your feet.

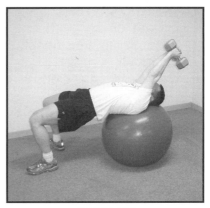

START

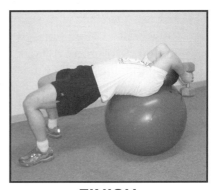

FINISH

DIFFICULTY -	H H H H
♂ STARTING WEIGHT - 25	
♀ STARTING WEIGHT - 12	

REVERSE GRIP LYING TRICEPS EXTENSION

MAJOR MUSCLES IN USE:
Triceps Brachii, Serratus Anterior

STARTING POSITION:
- Lie flat on a bench and hold a straight bar upwards at arms length directly above your forehead.
- Use an underhand grip with your hands about 6 – 8 inches apart.
- The angle between your arms and the floor should be approximately 80°.

EXERCISE MOVEMENT:
- While keeping your upper arms stationary, begin by bending your arms at the elbows and lowering the bar in a semicircular motion so that only the forearms are moving and the elbows remain in the same positions.
- Finish with the bar lightly touching the middle of the top of your head while keeping your elbows close together.
- Return the weight to the starting position while not allowing your elbows or your upper arms to move.

EXERCISE TECHNIQUE POINTS:
- Do not allow the barbell to lower so fast that you cannot control it.
- Do not allow your midsection to rise up causing excessive arching in your lower back.
- Your feet should remain on the floor and your hips and upper back should remain on the bench.
- Do not allow your elbows or upper arms to move excessively as you lower or raise the weight.

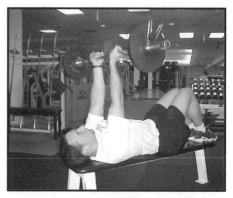

START

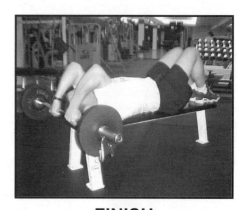

FINISH

DIFFICULTY -	H H H
♂	STARTING WEIGHT - 35
♀	STARTING WEIGHT - 20

CABLE LYING TRICEPS EXTENSION

MAJOR MUSCLES IN USE:
Triceps Brachii, Serratus Anterior

STARTING POSITION:
- Place the end of a flat bench approximately 1 – 2 feet from the bottom pulley.
- Lie on your back on the bench positioned so that your head is closest to the pulley. Support a short bar attached to the low pulley at arms length directly above your forehead. Your arms should be locked and supporting the weight.
- Use a comfortable overhand grip with your hands positioned about 8 – 12 inches apart.
- The angle between your arms and the floor should be approximately 80°.

EXERCISE MOVEMENT:
- While keeping your upper arms stationary, begin by bending the elbows and lowering the bar in a semicircular motion so that only the forearms are moving and the upper arms remain in the same position.
- Finish with the bar lightly touching the middle of the top of your head with your elbows staying close together as in the starting position.
- Return the weight to the starting position while not allowing your elbows or your upper arms to move.

EXERCISE TECHNIQUE POINTS:
- Do not allow the bar to lower so fast that you cannot control it.
- Do not allow your midsection to rise up causing excessive arching in your lower back.
- Your feet should remain on the floor and your hips and upper back should remain on the bench.
- Do not allow your elbows or your upper arms to move excessively as you lower or raise the weight.
- You may also perform this exercise one arm at a time with a single handle or with a reverse grip so that your palms are facing the floor.

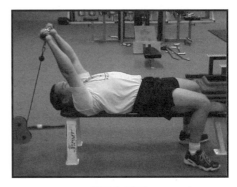
START

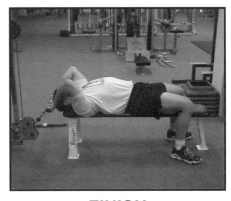
FINISH

DIFFICULTY -	H	H	H
♂ STARTING WEIGHT - 45			
♀ STARTING WEIGHT - 25			

LYING DUMBBELL TRICEPS EXTENSION

MAJOR MUSCLES IN USE:
Triceps Brachii, Serratus Anterior

STARTING POSITION:
- Before getting into position on the bench, grasp one end of a dumbbell with both hands. Either cup the bell with your hands or place your hands over top of one another at the very end of the bar.
- Lie flat on the bench with the dumbbell supported at arms length and positioned well past your forehead. Your arms should be locked to support the weight of the dumbbell.
- The angle between your arms and the floor should be approximately 60°.

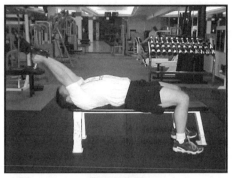

START

EXERCISE MOVEMENT:
- While keeping your upper arms stationary, bend at the elbow and lower the dumbbell in a semicircular motion so that only the forearms are moving and the elbows remain in the same position.
- Finish with one end of the dumbbell behind your head with your forearms touching the middle of the top of your head. Your elbows should remain close together as in the starting position.
- Return the weight to the starting position while not allowing your elbows or your upper arms to move.

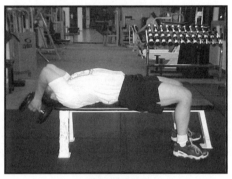

FINISH

EXERCISE TECHNIQUE POINTS:
- Do not allow the dumbbell to lower so fast that you cannot control it.
- Do not allow your midsection to rise up causing excessive arching in your lower back.
- Your feet should remain on the floor and your hips and upper back should remain on the bench.
- Do not allow your elbows or your upper arms to move excessively as you lower or raise the weight.
- For variety you may also choose to do this exercise with two dumbbells so that each dumbbell is held vertically in each hand.

DIFFICULTY -	H H H
♂ STARTING WEIGHT - 25	
♀ STARTING WEIGHT - 15	

TRICEPS EXERCISES

INCLINE LYING DUMBBELL TRICEPS EXTENSION

MAJOR MUSCLES IN USE:
 Triceps Brachii, Serratus Anterior

STARTING POSITION:
- Before getting into position, grasp two dumbbells.
- Lie on an incline bench positioned at approximately 40° to the floor and place the base of your skull at the top of the bench.
- Straighten your arms so that when your elbows are locked, they form an angle of approximately 60° - 70° to the floor.

EXERCISE MOVEMENT:
- While keeping your upper arms stationary, begin by bending at the elbow and lowering the dumbbells in a semicircular motion so that only the forearms are moving and the elbows remain in the same position.
- Finish with both ends of the dumbbells behind your head. Your hands should be touching both sides of your head. Your elbows should remain close together as in the starting position.
- Return the weight to the starting position while not allowing your elbows or your upper arms to move.

EXERCISE TECHNIQUE POINTS:
- Do not allow the dumbbells to lower so fast that you cannot control them.
- Do not allow your midsection to rise up causing excessive arching in your lower back.
- Your feet should remain on the floor and your hips and upper back should remain on the bench.
- Do not allow your elbows or your upper arms to move excessively as you lower or raise the weight.
- Try to keep the dumbbells from touching each other. However, this is not essential to proper form.

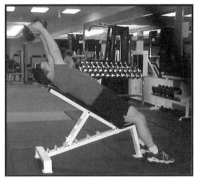

START

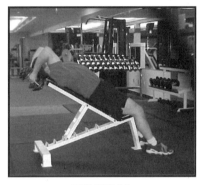

FINISH

DIFFICULTY -	⊢ ⊢ ⊢ ⊦
♂ STARTING WEIGHT - 15	
♀ STARTING WEIGHT - 8	

ONE ARM TRICEPS PUSHDOWN

MAJOR MUSCLES IN USE:
Triceps Brachii

STARTING POSITION:
- Standing with knees slightly bent in front of an overhead pulley machine, take an underhand grip on a single handle with one hand.
- Begin with your arm fully bent so that the handle is level with your mid-chest.
- Your upper arm should be tucked into your side and should not move during the exercise.
- A slight forward lean is allowed and may make the exercise more comfortable.

EXERCISE MOVEMENT:
- While keeping your upper arm stationary, begin by extending the arm in a semicircular motion so that only the forearm is moving and the elbow remains in the same position.
- At the mid-point of the movement, your arm should be bent at 90° with your forearm parallel to the floor.
- Finish with the handle beside your thigh and your arm fully extended.
- Return the weight to the starting position while not allowing your elbow to move forwards.

EXERCISE TECHNIQUE POINTS:
- Do not lean too far forward.
- Do not allow your elbow to move forward as you bring the weight back up.
- Do not allow the handle to rise higher than mid-chest.

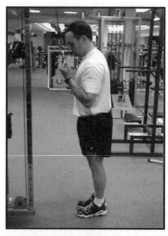

START

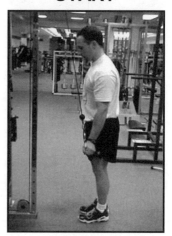

FINISH

DIFFICULTY -	H	H	H
♂ STARTING WEIGHT - 20			
♀ STARTING WEIGHT - 10			

TRICEPS EXERCISES

LYING TRICEPS HORIZONTAL EXTENSION

MAJOR MUSCLES IN USE:
Triceps Brachii, Serratus Anterior

STARTING POSITION:
* Lie on your back on a flat bench and, using both hands, hold a barbell at chest level with an overhand grip as wide as your chest.

EXERCISE MOVEMENT:
* Begin by extending your arms until they are horizontal to the floor. The bar should travel just above your chest and face as you straighten your arms outwards.
* The bar should follow a slight arc as you extend your arms your shoulders move naturally.
* At full extension, your arms should be straight and parallel to the floor. Reverse the motion so that you return the barbell back to chest level.

EXERCISE TECHNIQUE POINTS:
* Always keep your elbows as close together as possible.
* Do not allow your midsection to rise up causing excessive arching in your lower back.
* Your feet should remain on the floor and your hips and upper back should remain on the bench.

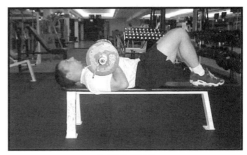

START

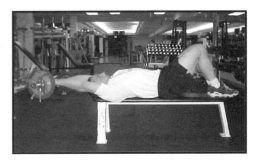

FINISH

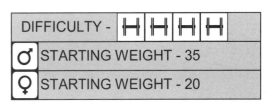

DIFFICULTY -	H H H H
♂ STARTING WEIGHT - 35	
♀ STARTING WEIGHT - 20	

LYING ONE ARM TRICEPS EXTENSION

MAJOR MUSCLES IN USE:
Triceps Brachii, Serratus Anterior

STARTING POSITION:
- Before getting into position on the bench, grasp one end of the dumbbell with one hand by either cupping the bell with your hand or by firmly grasping the bar at its very end.
- Lie on a flat bench with the dumbbell supported at arms length at an angle of about 60° to the floor. Your arm should be locked to support the weight of the dumbbell. If you wish you may use your other hand to stabilize the exercising arm.

EXERCISE MOVEMENT:
- While keeping your upper arm stationary, begin by bending at the elbow and lowering the dumbbell in a semicircular motion so that only the forearm is moving and the elbow remains in the same position.
- Finish with one end of the dumbbell beside your head.
- Return the weight to the starting position while not allowing your elbow or your upper arm to move.

EXERCISE TECHNIQUE POINTS:
- Do not allow the dumbbell to lower so fast that you cannot control it.
- Do not allow your midsection to rise up causing excessive arching in your lower back.
- Do not allow your elbow to point out as your triceps become tired.
- Do not allow your elbow or your upper arm to move excessively as you lower or raise the weight.

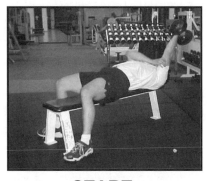

START

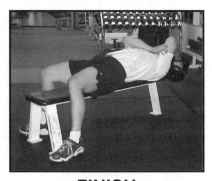

FINISH

DIFFICULTY -	⊢ ⊢ ⊢
♂ STARTING WEIGHT - 15	
♀ STARTING WEIGHT - 8	

ONE ARM SIDE TRICEPS EXTENSION

MAJOR MUSCLES IN USE:
Triceps Brachii, Serratus Anterior

STARTING POSITION:
- Before getting into position on the bench, grasp the middle of a dumbbell bar with one hand.
- Lie on your side on a flat bench with the dumbbell supported at arms length and with your arm positioned so that it is perpendicular to the floor. Your arm should be locked to support the weight of the dumbbell.

EXERCISE MOVEMENT:
- While keeping your upper arm stationary, begin by bending at the elbow and lower the dumbbell in a semicircular motion so that only the forearm is moving and the elbow remains at the same position.
- Finish with the dumbbell behind your head.
- Return the weight to the starting position while not allowing your elbow or your upper arm to move.

EXERCISE TECHNIQUE POINTS:
- Do not allow the dumbbell to lower so fast that you cannot control it.
- Do not allow your body to roll to one side in order to complete the repetitions.
- Do not allow your elbow to point downwards as you get tired.
- Do not allow your elbow or your upper arm to move excessively as you lower or raise the weight.

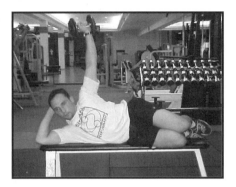

START

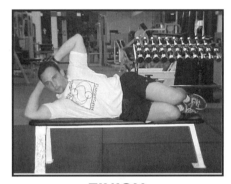

FINISH

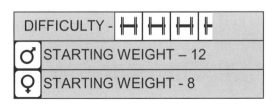

DIFFICULTY - H H H I-	
♂	STARTING WEIGHT – 12
♀	STARTING WEIGHT - 8

CROSS-BODY LYING ONE ARM TRICEPS EXTENSION

MAJOR MUSCLES IN USE:
Triceps Brachii, Serratus Anterior

STARTING POSITION:
- Before getting into position on the bench, grasp one end of the dumbbell with one hand by either cupping the bell with your hand or by firmly grasping the bar at its very end.
- Lie flat on the bench and hold the dumbbell at arms length directly above the shoulder.
- The palm of your hand should be facing towards your feet.

EXERCISE MOVEMENT:
- While keeping your upper arm stationary, begin by bending at the elbow and lower the dumbbell in a semicircular motion across your body so that only the forearm moves and the elbow remains in the same position.
- Finish with the dumbbell on the opposite side of your head.
- Return the weight to the starting position while not allowing your elbow or your upper arm to move.

EXERCISE TECHNIQUE POINTS:
- Do not allow the dumbbell to lower so fast that you cannot control it.
- Do not allow your torso to twist or your shoulder to come off the bench in order to lift the weight.
- Do not allow your elbow to point outwards as you become fatigued.
- Do not allow your elbow or your upper arm to move excessively as you lower or raise the weight.
- If you wish you can stabilize the exercising upper arm with your opposite hand to minimize any unwanted movement.

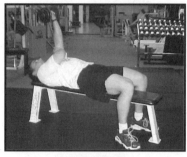

START

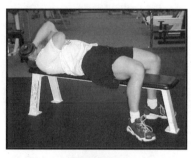

FINISH

DIFFICULTY -	H H H
♂ STARTING WEIGHT - 15	
♀ STARTING WEIGHT - 8	

CROSS BENCH TRICEPS EXTENSION

MAJOR MUSCLES IN USE:
Triceps Brachii, Serratus Anterior

STARTING POSITION:
- Before getting into position on the bench, grasp one end of the dumbbell with both hands. Either cup the bell with both hands or place your hands over top of one another at the very end of the bar.
- Lie across the narrow portion of a flat bench so that your upper shoulders, neck, and the base of your head are supporting your body weight. Your feet should be flat on the floor with your knees bent.
- Position the dumbbell so that it is supported at arms length directly above your forehead. Your arms should be straight and elbows locked to support the weight of the dumbbell.
- The angle between your arms and the floor should be approximately 70°.

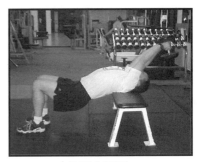

START

EXERCISE MOVEMENT:
- While keeping your upper arms stationary, begin by bending your elbows and lowering the dumbbell in a semicircular motion so that only the forearms are moving and the elbows remain in the same position.
- Finish with one end of the dumbbell behind your head with your hands touching the middle of the top of your head. Your elbows should remain as close together as they were in the starting position.
- Return the weight to the starting position while not allowing your elbows or your upper arms to move.

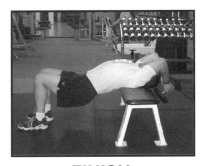

FINISH

EXERCISE TECHNIQUE POINTS:
- Do not allow the dumbbell to lower so fast that you cannot control it.
- Keep your hips low to the ground at all times in order to counter-act the weight of the dumbbell.
- Do not allow your elbows or your upper arms to move excessively as you lower or raise the weight.

DIFFICULTY -	� ⊢
♂ STARTING WEIGHT - 35	
♀ STARTING WEIGHT - 15	

TRICEPS EXERCISES 243

SEATED DUMBBELL TRICEPS EXTENSION

MAJOR MUSCLES IN USE:
Triceps Brachii, Serratus Anterior

STARTING POSITION:
- Sit on an exercise bench and tense your abdominal muscles.
- Position your hands on a dumbbell so that they are both at one end of the dumbbell and are either cupping the bell or are gripping the bar with one hand over top of the other.
- While keeping your hands in the same position, lift the dumbbell up so that it is directly above your head with your arms locked.
- If the weight is too heavy to lift into position with the correct hand placement, lift the dumbbell and place it on one of your shoulders. Now it will be easier to place your hands properly and lift it above your head.

EXERCISE MOVEMENT:
- While keeping your upper arms stationary, begin by bending at the elbow and lowering the dumbbell in a semicircular motion so that only the forearms are moving and the elbows remain in the same position.
- Finish with the dumbbell behind your head with your arms completely bent. Your elbows should remain close together during the exercise.
- Return the weight to the starting position while not allowing your elbows or your upper arms to move.

EXERCISE TECHNIQUE POINTS:
- Do not allow the dumbbell to lower so fast that you cannot control it.
- Be careful when lowering the dumbbell so that you do not hit the back of your head, neck or upper back.
- Do not bounce the dumbbell in the bottom position.

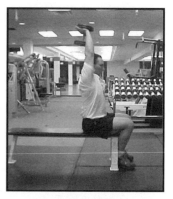

START

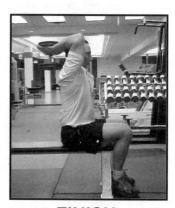

FINISH

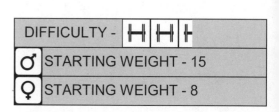

DIFFICULTY -	⊢ ⊢ ⊦
♂	STARTING WEIGHT - 15
♀	STARTING WEIGHT - 8

SEATED DOUBLE ARM DUMBBELL TRICEPS EXTENSION

MAJOR MUSCLES IN USE:
Triceps Brachii, Serratus Anterior

STARTING POSITION:
- Lie on an exercise bench inclined at approximately 45° and tense your abdominal muscles. Your head should be positioned level or slightly higher than the backrest of the bench.
- Grasp two dumbbells and position your hands vertically so that your thumb is pointing down towards the floor.
- While keeping your hands in the same position, lift the dumbbells up so that they are directly above your head with your arms locked.

EXERCISE MOVEMENT:
- While keeping your upper arms stationary, begin by bending at the elbows and lower the dumbbells in a semicircular motion so that only the forearms are moving while the elbows remain in the same position.
- Finish with the dumbbells behind your head with your arms completely bent. Your elbows should remain close together during the exercise.
- Return the weights to the starting position while not allowing your elbows or your upper arms to move.

EXERCISE TECHNIQUE POINTS:
- Do not allow the dumbbell to lower so fast that you cannot control it.
- Be careful when lowering the dumbbell so that you do not hit the back of your head, neck or upper back.
- Do not bounce the dumbbell in the bottom position.

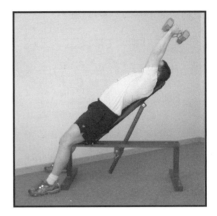

START

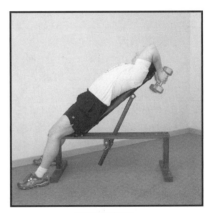

FINISH

DIFFICULTY -	⊢⊣ ⊢⊣ ⊢	
♂	STARTING WEIGHT - 15	
♀	STARTING WEIGHT - 8	

TRICEPS EXERCISES   245

ONE ARM TRICEPS EXTENSION

MAJOR MUSCLES IN USE:
Triceps Brachii, Serratus Anterior

STARTING POSITION:
- Sit down on a bench or if you prefer the standing version, stand with feet about shoulder width apart.
- Place one hand at one end of the dumbbell. Either cup the bell with your hand or grip the bar close to the bell.
- While keeping the same hand position, lift the dumbbell up so that it is directly above your head with your arm locked.

EXERCISE MOVEMENT:
- While keeping your upper arm stationary, begin by bending your elbow and lower the dumbbell behind your head. Only the forearm should move and the elbow remains in the same position.
- Finish with the dumbbell behind your head and with your arm completely bent. Your elbow should remain close to your head and pointing to the ceiling.
- Return the weight to the starting position while not allowing your elbow or your upper arm to move.

EXERCISE TECHNIQUE POINTS:
- Do not allow the dumbbell to lower so fast that you cannot control it.
- Take care when lowering the dumbbell so that you do not hit the back of your head, neck, or upper back.
- Do not bounce the dumbbell in the bottom position.

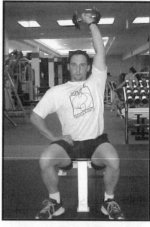

START

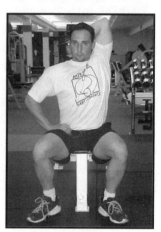

FINISH

DIFFICULTY - H H	
♂	STARTING WEIGHT - 15
♀	STARTING WEIGHT - 8

TRICEPS EXTENSION (FRENCH PRESS)

MAJOR MUSCLES IN USE:
Triceps Brachii, Serratus Anterior

STARTING POSITION:
- Sit on the edge of a bench or stand with feet about shoulder-width apart and your abdominal muscles tensed.
- Take an overhand grip approximately 6 – 8 inches apart using either an E-Z Curl bar or a standard straight bar. Lift the bar up above your head so that your arms are pointing straight up with your elbows locked.
- You may find the weight too heavy to lift into position while you are seated. If so, before you sit down, lift the weight up so that the bar is resting on your upper chest. Sit down and then press the weight up into position.

EXERCISE MOVEMENT:
- While keeping your upper arms stationary, begin by bending at the elbow and lower the barbell in a semicircular motion so that only the forearms move while the elbows remain in the same position.
- Finish with the bar behind your head and with your arms completely bent. Your elbows should remain as close together as in the starting position.
- Return the weight to the starting position while not allowing your elbows or your upper arms to move.

EXERCISE TECHNIQUE POINTS:
- Do not allow the bar to lower so fast that you cannot control it.
- Be careful when lowering the bar so that you do not hit the back of your head, neck or upper back.
- Do not bounce the bar in the bottom position.
- Keep your abdominal muscles tense and make sure you are careful not to arch your lower back excessively.
- You may also perform this exercise with a dumbbell held vertically in place of the bar.

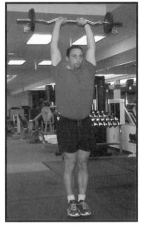

START

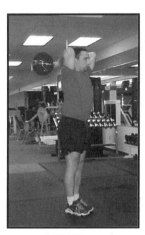

FINISH

DIFFICULTY -	H H H	
♂	STARTING WEIGHT - 35	
♀	STARTING WEIGHT - 20	

TRICEPS EXERCISES

STANDING CABLE TRICEPS EXTENSION

MAJOR MUSCLES IN USE:
Triceps Brachii, Serratus Anterior

STARTING POSITION:
- Grasp the rope handle, or short bar, attached to the low pulley with both hands and position yourself with your back towards the machine.
- Begin with your arms fully bent so that your hands are at the base of the back of your head and your elbows are close together.
- Bend your knees slightly and tense your abdominal muscles.

EXERCISE MOVEMENT:
- While keeping your upper arms stationary, begin by straightening your arms at the elbows and raising the rope handle or bar in a semicircular motion so that only the forearms are moving while the elbows remain in the same position.
- Finish with the handles or bar directly above your head and with your arms completely straight. Your elbows should remain as close together as in the starting position.
- Return the weight to the starting position while not allowing your elbows or your upper arms to move.

EXERCISE TECHNIQUE POINTS:
- Do not allow the bar or rope handle to lower so fast that you cannot control it.
- Be careful when lowering the bar that you do not hit the back of your head, neck or upper back.
- Do not bounce in the bottom part of the movement.
- Keep your abdominal muscles tense and make sure you are careful not to arch your lower back excessively.

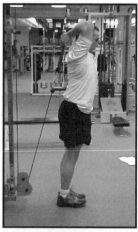

START

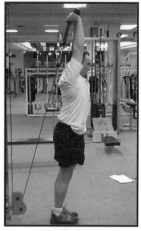

FINISH

DIFFICULTY -	H	H	H
♂ STARTING WEIGHT - 40			
♀ STARTING WEIGHT - 20			

TRICEPS EXERCISES

STANDING ONE ARM CABLE TRICEPS EXTENSION

MAJOR MUSCLES IN USE:
Triceps Brachii, Serratus Anterior

STARTING POSITION:
- Grasp the single handle attached to the low pulley with one hand and position yourself with your back towards the pulley machine.
- Begin with your arm fully bent so that your hand is behind your head at the base of your neck, palm up, with your elbow held close to the side of your head.
- Bend your knees slightly and tense your abdominal muscles.

EXERCISE MOVEMENT:
- While keeping your upper arm stationary, begin by straightening your arm at the elbow and raising the handle in a semicircular motion so that only the forearm is moving and the elbow remains in the same position.
- Finish with the handle directly above your head and your arm completely straight. Your elbow should remain close to your head as in the starting position.
- Return the weight to the starting position while not allowing your elbow or your upper arm to move.

EXERCISE TECHNIQUE POINTS:
- Do not allow the handle to lower so fast that you cannot control it.
- Be careful when lowering the handle that you do not hit the back of your head, neck or upper back.
- Do not bounce in the bottom part of the movement.
- Keep your abdominal muscles tensed and make sure you are careful not to arch your lower back excessively.

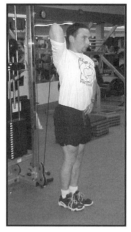

START

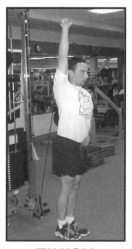

FINISH

DIFFICULTY -	H H H	
♂	STARTING WEIGHT - 10	
♀	STARTING WEIGHT - 5	

TRICEPS EXERCISES

TRICEPS KICKBACKS

MAJOR MUSCLES IN USE:

Triceps Brachii

STARTING POSITION:

- Position yourself on a bench so that one knee and one hand (from the same side of the body) are supporting your body on the bench. The other foot should be placed on the floor with the other hand grasping a dumbbell.
- Bend your arm at 90° so that your upper arm is parallel to the floor and your forearm is perpendicular to the floor. Your elbow should be directly at your side and held close to your torso.
- Your back should be flat and shoulders square with the floor.

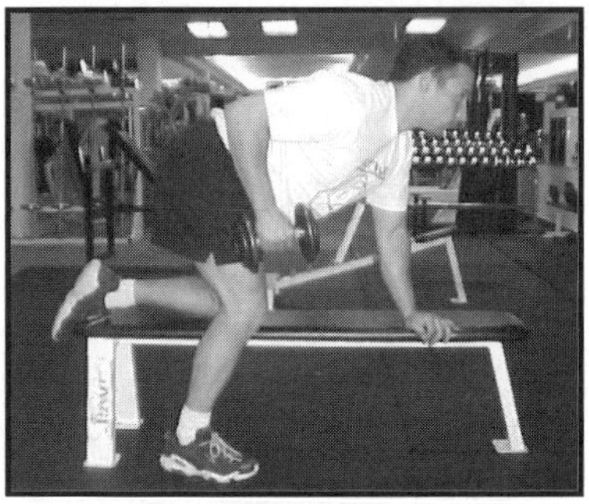

START

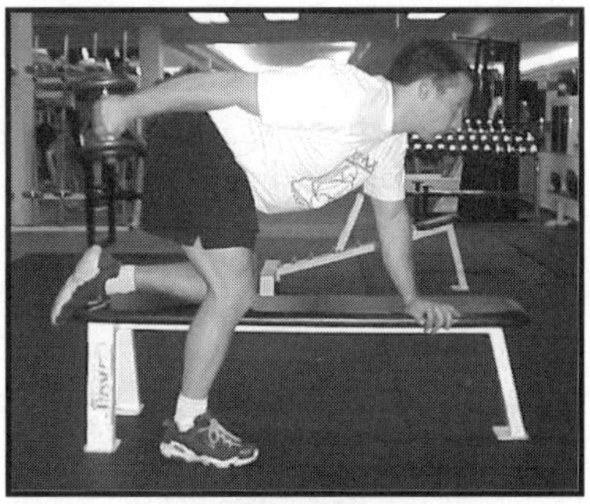

FINISH

EXERCISE MOVEMENT:

- While keeping your upper arm stationary and your back flat, straighten your arm by bending at the elbow and lift the weight up along an arcing path. Make sure you keep your elbow tucked in close to your side.
- Extend your arm until it is as straight as possible. Reverse the motion by lowering the dumbbell back along the same path that it was raised.

EXERCISE TECHNIQUE POINTS:

- Keep your chest high so that your upper back is flat with a slight arch in your lower back.
- Do not allow yourself to sway or twist excessively when performing your repetitions. Be careful of twisting the shoulders excessively as this can put unnecessary strain on your back muscles.
- Make sure you straighten the arm as much as possible while keeping your elbow close to your torso.
- Make sure to keep your upper arm stationary.

DIFFICULTY -

♂ STARTING WEIGHT - 12

♀ STARTING WEIGHT - 8

DOUBLE TRICEPS KICKBACKS

MAJOR MUSCLES IN USE:
Triceps Brachii

STARTING POSITION:
- Bend your knees slightly and bend forward at the waist so that your back is flat and parallel to the ground. Grasp two dumbbells and position your hands facing each other.
- Bend both your arms at 90° so that your upper arms are parallel to the floor and your forearms are perpendicular to the floor. Your elbows should be directly at your sides and held close to your torso.
- Your back should be flat and shoulders square with the floor.

EXERCISE MOVEMENT:
- While keeping your upper arms stationary and your back flat, straighten your arms by bending at the elbows and lift the weight up along an arcing path. Make sure you keep your elbows tucked in close to your sides.
- Extend your arms until they are as straight as possible. Reverse the motion by lowering the dumbbells back along the same path that they were raised. Your hands should return to the same place as when you began.

EXERCISE TECHNIQUE POINTS:
- Keep your chest high so that your upper back is flat with a slight arch in your lower back.
- Do not allow yourself to sway or twist excessively when performing your repetitions. Be careful of twisting the shoulders excessively as this can put unnecessary strain on your back muscles.
- Make sure you straighten the arms as much as possible while keeping your elbows close to your torso.
- Make sure to keep your upper arms stationary.

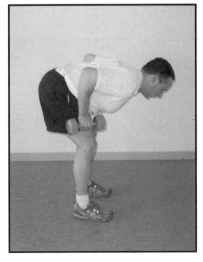

START

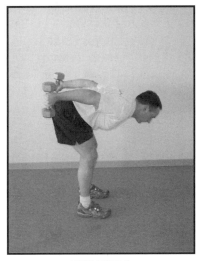

FINISH

DIFFICULTY -	⊢⊣ ⊢⊣ ⊢
♂ STARTING WEIGHT - 12	
♀ STARTING WEIGHT - 8	

CABLE TRICEPS KICKBACKS

MAJOR MUSCLES IN USE:

Triceps Brachii

STARTING POSITION:
- Face the front of the low pulley machine.
- Bend your knees slightly and bend forward at the waist so that your back is flat and parallel to the ground.
- Grasp the single handle attached to the cable and bend your arm at 90° so that your upper arm is parallel to the floor and your forearm is perpendicular to the floor.
- Your elbow should be at your side and held close to your torso. Your palm should be facing backwards with the front of your hand facing the machine.

EXERCISE MOVEMENT:
- While keeping your upper arm stationary and your back flat, straighten your arm by bending at the elbow and lift the weight up in an arcing motion. Make sure you keep your elbow tucked in close to your side.
- Extend your forearm arm backwards until it is as straight as possible. Reverse the motion by lowering the dumbbell back along the same path that it was raised so that your hand returns to the same place as when you began.

EXERCISE TECHNIQUE POINTS:
- Keep your chest high so that your upper back is flat with a slight arch in your lower back.
- Do not allow yourself to sway or twist excessively when performing your repetitions. Be careful of twisting the shoulders excessively as this can put unnecessary strain on your back muscles.
- Make sure you straighten the arm as much as possible while keeping your elbow close to your torso.
- Make sure you keep your upper arm stationary.
- You may also choose to use one side of a rope handle for variety.

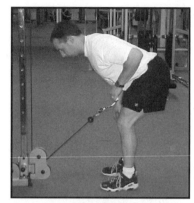

START

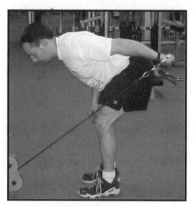

FINISH

DIFFICULTY -	H H H
♂ STARTING WEIGHT - 30	
♀ STARTING WEIGHT - 15	

TRICEPS EXERCISES

TRICEPS DIPS

MAJOR MUSCLES IN USE:

Triceps Brachii, Anterior Deltoid, Pectoralis Major

STARTING POSITION:

- Support yourself on the parallel bars of the dip station gripping the bars with your palms facing each other. Lock your arms to support your weight for now.
- Make sure you try to keep your torso as upright as possible by bringing your knees forward. In order to focus more on the triceps muscles, keep the elbows tucked in close to your sides. It may be necessary for you to bend your knees at 90° so that your feet will clear the floor.

EXERCISE MOVEMENT:

- While keeping your upper body vertical, descend into the bottom of the motion until your upper arms become parallel to the floor. You should feel a stretch in the shoulder, triceps, and chest muscles.
- Once reaching the bottom, immediately reverse the motion and push yourself up and back to the starting position. It is important not to pause at the bottom.

EXERCISE TECHNIQUE POINTS:

- Remember to try and stay as upright as possible.
- Keep your elbows tucked in close to your sides. This will work the triceps muscle more directly.
- Do not bounce at the bottom portion of the exercise.
- Do not allow your upper arm to go much beyond a position that is parallel with the floor since doing so will put added stress on your elbows and shoulders.
- You may also wish to add weight by using a specially designed belt that goes around your waist or by holding a dumbbell between your feet.

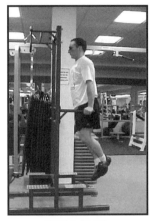

START

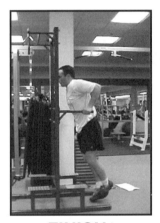

FINISH

DIFFICULTY -	⊢ ⊢	
♂	STARTING WEIGHT – no weight	
♀	STARTING WEIGHT – no weight	

BENCH DIPS

MAJOR MUSCLES IN USE:
Triceps Brachii, Anterior Deltoid

STARTING POSITION:
- Position yourself perpendicular between two benches placed about 3 feet apart and parallel to each other. Your torso should be perpendicular to the floor. Support yourself on the heels of your hands on one of the benches with your fingers facing forward. Place your heels on the other bench.
- With your arms locked, you should look like the letter 'L' suspended between the two benches so that the angle between your outstretched legs and your torso is approximately 90°. In order to focus more on the triceps muscles, keep the elbows tucked in close to your sides.

EXERCISE MOVEMENT:
- While keeping your upper body vertical, descend into the bottom of the motion so that your upper arms become parallel to the floor. You should feel a stretch in the shoulder, triceps, and chest muscles.
- Once you reach the bottom, immediately reverse the motion and push yourself back to the starting position. It is important not to pause at the bottom.

EXERCISE TECHNIQUE POINTS:
- Remember to try and stay as vertical as possible.
- Keep your elbows in close to your sides so that you work the triceps muscles.
- Do not bounce at the bottom portion of the exercise.
- Do not allow your upper arms to go much beyond a line that is parallel with the floor as this will put added stress on your elbows and shoulders.
- In order to make the exercise more difficult, you may wish to add a weight to your lap. In order to make it less difficult, place your feet on the ground.

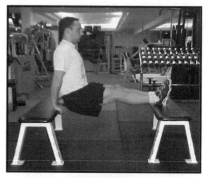

START

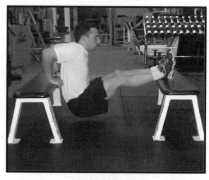

FINISH

DIFFICULTY -	H	H
♂ STARTING WEIGHT – no weight		
♀ STARTING WEIGHT – no weight		

BICEPS EXERCISES

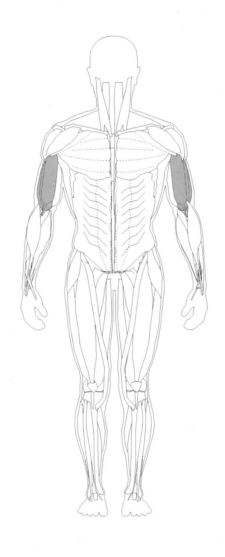

BARBELL CURLS

MAJOR MUSCLES IN USE:
Biceps Brachii, Brachialis

STARTING POSITION:
- Stand with your knees slightly bent and feet about shoulder width apart.
- With your arms hanging straight at your sides hold the bar using an underhand grip about chest width apart.

EXERCISE MOVEMENT:
- While keeping your upper arms stationary, begin by allowing your elbows to bend as you lift the weight in a semicircular motion.
- At the midpoint of the movement, your arms should be bent with your forearms parallel to the floor and your upper arms perpendicular to the floor.
- Finish with the barbell at shoulder level. Your upper arms should remain perpendicular to the floor.
- Return the weight to the starting position while not allowing your elbows to move backwards.
- Before you start another repetition, your arms should be straight.

EXERCISE TECHNIQUE POINTS:
- Do not sway your torso back and forth.
- Do not allow your elbows to move backwards or forwards as you lift the weight up.
- Maintain good posture with your back straight at all times.
- Do not bend your knees or "jump" the weight up to complete a repetition.

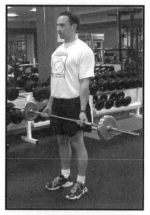

START

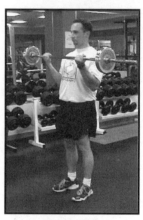

FINISH

DIFFICULTY -	⊢⊣
♂ STARTING WEIGHT - 55	
♀ STARTING WEIGHT - 25	

BICEPS EXERCISES

E-Z BAR CURLS

MAJOR MUSCLES IN USE:
Biceps Brachii, Brachialis

STARTING POSITION:
- Stand with your knees slightly bent and feet about shoulder width apart.
- Grasp an E-Z curl bar with an underhand grip so that your thumbs are higher than your smallest fingers and your hands are about 6 – 10 inches apart.
- Arms should be hanging straight at your sides with the bar resting on your upper thighs.

EXERCISE MOVEMENT:
- While keeping your upper arms stationary, begin by bending at the elbows and lifting the weight upwards following the natural curve of your arm's movement.
- At the midpoint in the motion, your elbows should be bent at 90° with your forearms parallel to the floor and your upper arms perpendicular to the floor.
- Finish with the barbell at shoulder level. Your upper arms should remain perpendicular to the floor.
- Return the weight to the starting position while not allowing your elbows to move backwards.
- Before you start another repetition, your arms should be straight.

EXERCISE TECHNIQUE POINTS:
- Do not sway your torso back and forth.
- Do not allow your elbows to move backwards or forwards as you lift the weight.
- Maintain good posture with your back straight at all times.
- Do not bend your knees or "jump" the weight up to complete a repetition.
- If you wish, you may experiment with the kind of grip you are using to hold the bar. You may choose either a close grip position or a wide grip position.

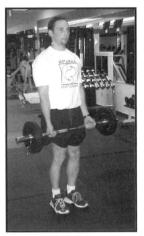

START

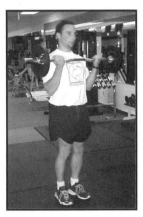

FINISH

DIFFICULTY -	H	
♂	STARTING WEIGHT - 55	
♀	STARTING WEIGHT - 25	

BICEPS EXERCISES   257

DUMBBELL CURLS

MAJOR MUSCLES IN USE:
Biceps Brachii, Brachialis

STARTING POSITION:
- Stand with knees slightly bent and feet about shoulder width apart.
- Arms should hang straight at your sides. The dumbbells should be beside your upper thighs.
- Take an underhand grip on each dumbbell so that your palms are facing forward.

EXERCISE MOVEMENT:
- While keeping your upper arms stationary, begin by bending your arms at the elbows and lift the dumbbells upwards following a semicircular motion.
- At midpoint in the motion, your elbows should be bent at 90° with your forearms parallel to the floor and your upper arms perpendicular to the floor.
- Finish the movement with the dumbbells in front of your shoulders while your upper arms remain perpendicular to the floor. The backs of your hands are now facing directly forward.
- Return the weight to the starting position while not allowing your elbows to move backwards.
- Before starting another repetition, your arms should be straight.

EXERCISE TECHNIQUE POINTS:
- Do not sway your torso back and forth.
- Do not allow your elbows to move backwards or forwards as you lift the weight up.
- Maintain good posture with your back straight at all times.
- Do not bend your knees or "jump" the weight up to complete a repetition.

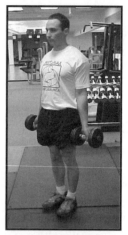

START

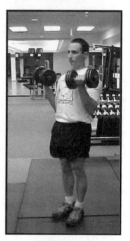

FINISH

DIFFICULTY - ⊞		
♂	STARTING WEIGHT - 15	
♀	STARTING WEIGHT - 10	

BICEPS EXERCISES

SEATED DUMBBELL CURLS

MAJOR MUSCLES IN USE:
Biceps Brachii, Brachialis

STARTING POSITION:
- Sit on the end of a bench with your chest held high and your feet together.
- Hold a dumbbell in each hand using an underhand grip so that your palms are facing forward.
- Arms should hang straight at your sides with the dumbbells resting below the level of the bench.

EXERCISE MOVEMENT:
- While keeping your upper arms stationary, begin by bending at the elbows and lifting the dumbbells upwards following the natural curve of your arm's movement.
- At midpoint in the motion, your elbows should be bent at 90° with your forearms parallel to the floor and your upper arms perpendicular to the floor.
- Finish with the dumbbells held in front of your shoulders while your upper arms remain perpendicular to the floor. At this point, the backs of your hands should face forward.
- Return the weight to the starting position while not allowing your elbows to move backwards.
- Before starting another repetition, your arms should be straight.

EXERCISE TECHNIQUE POINTS:
- Do not sway your torso back and forth.
- Do not allow your elbows to move backwards or forwards as you lift the weight up.
- Maintain good posture with your back straight at all times.
- Do not lean to one side to complete a repetition.
- You may also perform this exercise with a thumbs up position or "hammer" grip.

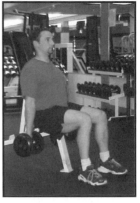

START

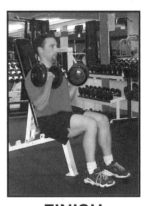

FINISH

DIFFICULTY -	⊢∣	
♂	STARTING WEIGHT - 15	
♀	STARTING WEIGHT - 10	

HAMMER CURLS

MAJOR MUSCLES IN USE:
   Biceps Brachii, Brachialis

STARTING POSITION:
- Stand with your knees slightly bent and feet close together. Hold a dumbbell in each hand.
- Arms should hang straight at your sides with the dumbbells resting beside your upper thighs.
- Hold the dumbbells so that your palms are facing in towards your thighs.

EXERCISE MOVEMENT:
- While keeping your upper arms stationary, begin by bending at the elbows and lifting the dumbbells upwards following the natural curve of your arm's motion.
- At the midpoint in the motion, your elbows should be bent at 90° with your forearms parallel to the floor and your upper arms perpendicular to the floor. Your palms should be facing each other throughout the whole range of motion.
- Finish with the dumbbells in front of your shoulders while your upper arms remain perpendicular to the floor.
- Return the weight to the starting position while not allowing your elbows to move backwards. Before you start another repetition, your arms should be straight.

EXERCISE TECHNIQUE POINTS:
- Do not sway your torso back and forth.
- Do not allow your elbows to move backwards or forwards as you lift the weight.
- Maintain good posture with your back straight at all times.
- Do not bend your knees or "jump" the weight up to complete a repetition.

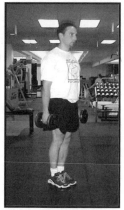

START

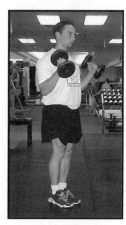

FINISH

DIFFICULTY -	⊢	
♂	STARTING WEIGHT - 15	
♀	STARTING WEIGHT - 10	

ALTERNATING DUMBBELL CURLS

MAJOR MUSCLES IN USE:
Biceps Brachii, Brachialis

STARTING POSITION:
- Stand with your knees slightly bent and feet about shoulder width apart. Hold a dumbbell in each hand.
- Arms should hang straight at your sides with the dumbbells resting beside your upper thighs.
- Take an overhand grip on each bar so that your palms are facing your upper thighs.

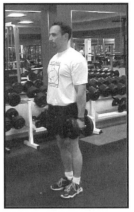

START

EXERCISE MOVEMENT:
- While keeping your upper arms stationary, begin by bending only one arm at the elbow and lifting the dumbbell in a semicircular motion. The other arm should remain straight.
- As soon as the dumbbell clears your thigh, twist your hand up so that your palm is facing up.
- At the midpoint in the motion, your elbow should be bent at 90° to your body with your forearm parallel to the floor and your upper arm perpendicular to the floor.
- Finish with the dumbbell in front of your shoulder and your upper arm still perpendicular to the floor. The back of your hand should face directly forward.
- Return the weight to the starting position while not allowing your elbow to move.
- Follow the same set of instructions for the other arm.
- Before you start another repetition, your arm should once again be straight.

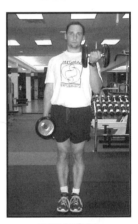

FINISH

EXERCISE TECHNIQUE POINTS:
- Do not sway your torso back and forth.
- Do not allow your elbow to move backwards or forwards as you lift the weight up.
- Maintain good posture with your back straight at all times.
- Do not bend your knees or "jump" the weight up to complete a repetition.
- Do not lean from side to side in order to complete a repetition.

DIFFICULTY -	⊢∣⊦	
♂	STARTING WEIGHT - 15	
♀	STARTING WEIGHT - 10	

ZOTTMAN CURL

MAJOR MUSCLES IN USE:
  Biceps Brachii, Brachialis

STARTING POSITION:
- Stand with your knees slightly bent and feet about shoulder width apart.
- Hold a dumbbell in each hand taking an underhand grip so that your palms are facing forwards.
- Arms should hang straight at your sides with the dumbbells resting beside your upper thighs (as shown in the pictures on this page).

EXERCISE MOVEMENT:
- While keeping your upper arms stationary, begin by bending only one arm at the elbow and lift the dumbbell in a semicircular motion. The other arm should remain straight.
- At midpoint in the motion, your elbows should be bent at 90° with your forearms parallel to the floor and your upper arms perpendicular to the floor.
- Finish with the dumbbell in front of your shoulders and your upper arm still perpendicular to the floor and the back of your hand facing directly forward.
- As you lower the weight back to the starting position, twist your hand around so that your palm is facing forward and then downward.
- As you lower the weight with your palm down, your other arm should be just starting to lift the weight up as the first arm had previously done.

EXERCISE TECHNIQUE POINTS:
- Do not sway your torso back and forth.
- Do not allow your elbow to move backwards or forwards as you lift the weight up.
- Maintain good posture with your back straight at all times.
- Do not bend your knees or "jump" the weight up to complete a repetition.
- Do not lean from side to side in order to complete a repetition.
- Make sure your arm straightens before starting another repetition.
- Make sure you keep your elbows in close to your sides.

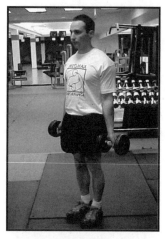

START

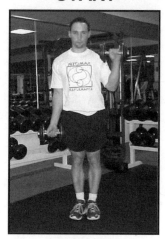

FINISH

DIFFICULTY -	H H H H
♂ STARTING WEIGHT - 15	
♀ STARTING WEIGHT - 8	

BICEPS EXERCISES

PRONATING DUMBBELL CURLS

MAJOR MUSCLES IN USE:
Biceps Brachii, Brachialis

STARTING POSITION:
- Stand with your knees slightly bent and feet about shoulder width apart. Hold a dumbbell in each hand.
- Arms should hang straight at your sides with the dumbbells resting beside your upper thighs.
- Hold the dumbbells so that your palms are facing in towards your thighs.

EXERCISE MOVEMENT:
- While keeping your upper arms stationary, begin by bending at the elbows and lifting the dumbbells upwards following the natural curve of your arms' motion.
- As soon as the dumbbells clear your thighs, twist your hands outwards so that your palms are now facing up.
- At midpoint in the motion, your elbows should be bent at 90° with your forearms parallel to the floor and your upper arms still perpendicular to the floor.
- Finish with the dumbbells in front of your shoulders with your upper arms remaining perpendicular to the floor and the backs of your hands facing directly forward.
- Lower the weights back to the starting position along the same path that you lifted them while not allowing your elbows to move backwards.
- Before starting another repetition, your arms should once again be straight.

EXERCISE TECHNIQUE POINTS:
- Do not sway your torso back and forth.
- Do not allow your elbows to move backwards or forwards as you lift the weight up.
- Maintain good posture with your back straight at all times.
- Do not bend your knees or "jump" the weight up to complete a repetition.
- Make sure your palms are facing upwards at the mid-point in the movement.

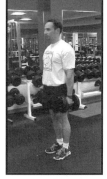

START

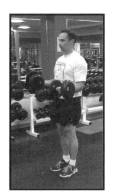

MIDDLE

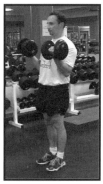

FINISH

DIFFICULTY -	⊢⊣ ⊢⊣ ⊢	
♂	STARTING WEIGHT - 15	
♀	STARTING WEIGHT - 10	

INCLINE CURLS

MAJOR MUSCLES IN USE:
 Biceps Brachii, Brachialis

STARTING POSITION:
- Sit with your knees together on an incline bench that is inclined back to about an angle of 60° to the floor.
- Arms should hang straight down perpendicular to the floor.
- Take an underhand grip so that your palms are facing forward.

EXERCISE MOVEMENT:
- While keeping your upper arms stationary, begin by bending your arms at the elbows and lifting the dumbbells upwards following the natural curve of your arm movement.
- At midpoint in the motion, your elbows should be bent at 90° with your forearms parallel to the floor and your upper arms perpendicular to the floor.
- Finish with the dumbbells in front of your shoulders, your upper arms still perpendicular to the floor, and the backs of your hands facing directly forward.
- Return the weights to the starting position while not allowing your elbows to move backwards.
- Before you start another repetition your arms should be straight.

EXERCISE TECHNIQUE POINTS:
- Do not allow your back to arch in order to complete a repetition.
- Do not allow your elbows to move forward as you lift the weight.
- Maintain good posture with your chest held high.
- Do not swing the weight in order to complete a repetition.
- You may also perform this exercise with a thumb up position or "hammer" grip.

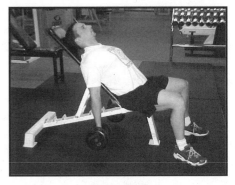

START

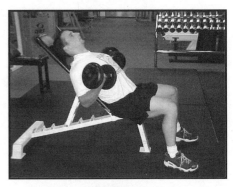

FINISH

DIFFICULTY -	⊢ ⊢	
♂	STARTING WEIGHT - 15	
♀	STARTING WEIGHT - 8	

BICEPS EXERCISES

CABLE CURLS

MAJOR MUSCLES IN USE:
Biceps Brachii, Brachialis

STARTING POSITION:
- Stand with your feet about shoulder width apart. Grasp a short bar that is attached to the low pulley of a cable machine and take an underhand grip about chest-width apart.
- Allow your arms to straighten so that the bar is just above mid-thigh level.
- With your knees slightly bent, straighten your back and shoulders by holding your chest high.

EXERCISE MOVEMENT:
- While keeping your upper arms stationary, bend at the elbows and lift the bar up following the natural motion or your arm.
- At midpoint in the motion your elbows should be bent at 90° with your forearms parallel to the floor and your upper arms perpendicular to the floor.
- Finish with the bar in front of your chest. Your upper arms should remain perpendicular to the floor and the backs of your hands should face directly forward.
- Return the bar to the starting position while not allowing your elbows to move backwards.
- Before you start another repetition, your arms should be straight.

EXERCISE TECHNIQUE POINTS:
- Do not sway your torso back and forth.
- Do not allow your elbow to move backwards or forwards as you lift the weight up.
- Maintain good posture with your back straight at all times.
- Do not bend your knees or "jump" the weight up to complete a repetition.

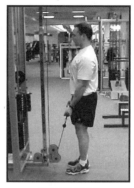

START

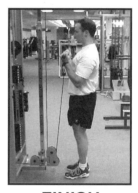

FINISH

DIFFICULTY -	H	
♂	STARTING WEIGHT - 45	
♀	STARTING WEIGHT - 25	

BICEPS EXERCISES

HAMMER CABLE CURLS

MAJOR MUSCLES IN USE:
Biceps Brachii, Brachialis

STARTING POSITION:
- Stand with feet about shoulder width apart. Grasp a rope handle that is attached to the low pulley of a cable machine and take a grip so that the palms of your hands are facing each other.
- Allow your arms to straighten so that the rope ends are just above mid-thigh level.
- With your knees slightly bent, straighten your back and shoulders by holding your chest high.

EXERCISE MOVEMENT:
- While keeping your upper arms stationary, bend at the elbows and lift the handle up following the natural motion of your arm.
- At midpoint in the motion your elbows should be bent at 90° with your forearms parallel to the floor and your upper arms perpendicular to the floor.
- Finish with the rope ends in front of your chest. Your upper arms should remain perpendicular to the floor and the palms of your hands should face each other.
- Return the bar to the starting position while not allowing your elbows to move backwards.
- Before you start another repetition, your arms should be straight.

EXERCISE TECHNIQUE POINTS:
- Do not sway your torso back and forth.
- Do not allow your elbows to move backwards or forwards as you lift the weight up.
- Maintain good posture with your back straight at all times.
- Do not bend your knees or "jump" the weight up to complete a repetition.

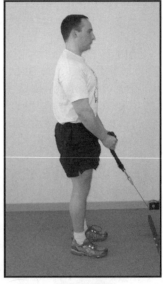

START

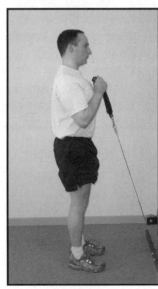

FINISH

DIFFICULTY -	H	
♂	STARTING WEIGHT - 45	
♀	STARTING WEIGHT - 25	

ONE ARM CABLE CURLS

MAJOR MUSCLES IN USE:
Biceps Brachii, Brachialis

STARTING POSITION:
- Stand with feet about shoulder width apart. Grasp a single handle with an underhand grip attached to the cable of a low pulley machine.
- With your arm straight, hold the handle beside your upper thigh.
- Bend at the knees slightly and straighten your back by keeping your chest held high.
- If you wish, you may stabilize your upper body by hanging onto the machine.

EXERCISE MOVEMENT:
- While keeping your upper arm stationary, begin by bending at the elbow and lift the handle up following a semicircular path.
- At midpoint in the motion your elbow should be bent at 90° with your forearm parallel to the floor and your upper arm perpendicular to the floor.
- Finish with the handle in front of your shoulder. Your upper arm should remain perpendicular to the floor and the back of your hand should face forward.
- Return the weight to the starting position while not allowing your elbow to move backwards.
- Before you start another repetition your arm should be straight.

EXERCISE TECHNIQUE POINTS:
- Do not sway your torso back and forth.
- Do not allow your elbows to move backwards or forwards as you lift the weight.
- Maintain good posture with your back straight at all times.
- Do not bend your knees or "jump" the weight up to complete a repetition.
- You may also perform this exercise with a thumb up position or hammer grip by using one side of a rope handle.

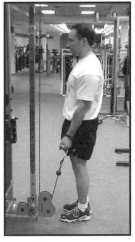

START

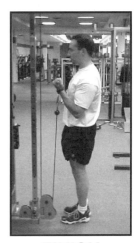

FINISH

DIFFICULTY -	⊢⊣ �	
♂	STARTING WEIGHT - 20	
♀	STARTING WEIGHT - 10	

STANDING ONE ARM STRETCH CABLE CURLS

MAJOR MUSCLES IN USE:
    Biceps Brachii, Brachialis

STARTING POSITION:
- Stand about 3 - 4 feet in front of a low pulley machine with your back facing the machine. Take an underhand grip on a single handle attached to the cable from the machine.
- Place one foot in front of the other and allow your exercising arm to straighten. Your arm should be pulled back so that your hand is at least 6 inches behind your hip.
- Straighten your back and shoulders by holding your chest up.

EXERCISE MOVEMENT:
- While keeping your upper arm stationary, begin by bending at the elbow and pull the handle forwards and up following the natural movement of your arm.
- Finish the movement with the handle just below your shoulder. Your upper arm should remain at an angle to the floor.
- Return the weight to the starting position while not allowing your elbow to move forwards or backwards.
- Before you start another repetition, your arm should once again be straight.

EXERCISE TECHNIQUE POINTS:
- Do not sway your torso back and forth.
- Do not allow your elbow to move backwards or forwards as you lift the weight.
- Maintain good posture with your back straight at all times. You may also perform this exercise with a thumb up position or hammer grip using one side of a rope handle.

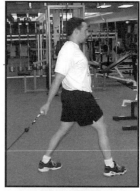

START

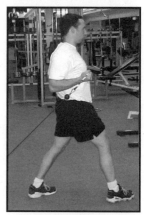

FINISH

DIFFICULTY -	H	H	
♂	STARTING WEIGHT - 20		
♀	STARTING WEIGHT - 10		

BICEPS EXERCISES

BARBELL PREACHER CURLS

MAJOR MUSCLES IN USE:
Biceps Brachii, Brachialis

STARTING POSITION:
- Sit at a preacher bench so that the bottom portion of your chest is level with the top of the bench.
- Take an underhand grip on the bar and place your hands about shoulder width apart.

EXERCISE MOVEMENT:
- Keep your upper body stationary as you lift the bar upwards and along a semicircular path towards your chin.
- Finish with your forearms perpendicular to the floor and the barbell at face level.
- Lower the weight back along the same path that you raised it. Stop just before your arms straighten. From this position repeat the motion again for the desired number of repetitions.

EXERCISE TECHNIQUE POINTS:
- Do not sway your torso back and forth.
- Do not allow your elbows to rise off the bench.
- Maintain good posture with your back straight at all times.
- Do not allow your arms to straighten all the way. Always keep a slight bend at the elbows in order to protect them from injury.
- Do not allow yourself to rise from the seat during the exercise.

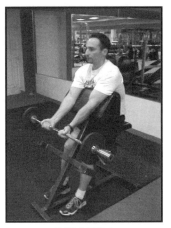

START

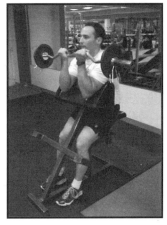

FINISH

DIFFICULTY -	⊢┤ ╟	
♂	STARTING WEIGHT - 40	
♀	STARTING WEIGHT - 20	

DUMBBELL PREACHER CURLS

MAJOR MUSCLES IN USE:
Biceps Brachii, Brachialis

STARTING POSITION:
- Sit at a preacher bench so that the bottom portion of your chest is level with the top of the bench.
- Grasp a pair of dumbbells with an underhand grip and space your hands about shoulder width apart.

EXERCISE MOVEMENT:
- While keeping your torso stationary, lift the dumbbells up along a semicircular path towards your chin.
- Finish the movement with your forearms perpendicular to the floor and the dumbbells about level with your face.
- Lower the weight back along the same path that you lifted them, but make sure to stop just before your arms straighten. From this point begin the exercise again.

EXERCISE TECHNIQUE POINTS:
- Do not sway your torso back and forth.
- Do not allow your elbows to rise off the bench.
- Maintain good posture with your back straight at all times.
- Do not allow your arms to straighten all the way. Always keep a slight bend in the elbows in order to protect them from injury.
- Do not allow yourself to rise from the seat during the motion.
- You may also perform this exercise with a thumb up position or hammer grip.

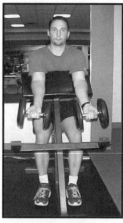

START

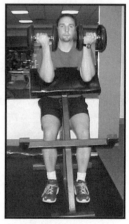

FINISH

DIFFICULTY -	⊢⊣ ⊢⊣	
♂	STARTING WEIGHT - 15	
♀	STARTING WEIGHT - 10	

BICEPS EXERCISES

ONE ARM DUMBBELL PREACHER CURL

MAJOR MUSCLES IN USE:
Biceps Brachii, Brachialis

STARTING POSITION:
- Sit at a preacher bench so that the bottom portion of your chest is level with the top of the bench.
- Take an underhand grip on a dumbbell and place the dumbbell so that it is below and in line with your shoulder. Your other arm, if you wish, can rest across the top of the bench.

EXERCISE MOVEMENT:
- While keeping your torso stationary, begin by lifting the dumbbell in a semicircular motion towards your chin.
- Finish with your forearm perpendicular to the floor and the dumbbell at mid-face level.
- Lower the weight back along the same path that you lifted it, but stop just before your arm straightens. From this position, begin the repetition again.

EXERCISE TECHNIQUE POINTS:
- Do not sway your torso back and forth.
- Do not allow your elbow to rise off the bench.
- Maintain good posture with your back straight at all times.
- Do not allow your arm to straighten all the way. Always keep a slight bend in the elbow in order to protect it from injury.
- Keep yourself seated. Do not allow yourself to rise from the seat during the motion.
- You may also perform this exercise with a thumb up position or hammer grip.

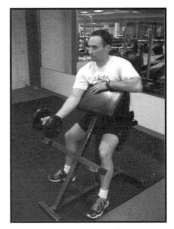

START

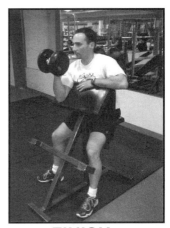

FINISH

DIFFICULTY - ⊢⊣ ⊢⊣	
♂ STARTING WEIGHT - 15	
♀ STARTING WEIGHT - 10	

CABLE PREACHER CURL

MAJOR MUSCLES IN USE:
Biceps Brachii, Brachialis

STARTING POSITION:
- Sit at a preacher bench so that the bottom portion of your chest is level with and pushed in tightly against the top of the bench.
- Take an underhand grip on a short bar that is attached to the low pulley of the pulley machine. Space your hands about shoulder width apart.

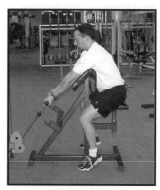

START

EXERCISE MOVEMENT:
- While keeping your torso stationary, begin by lifting the bar up along a semicircular path towards your chin.
- Finish with your forearms perpendicular to the floor and the bar level with your face.
- Lower the weight back along the same path that you lifted it but stop just before your arms straighten. Repeat the motion for the desired number of repetitions.

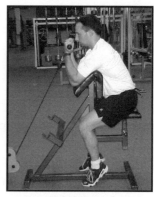

FINISH

EXERCISE TECHNIQUE POINTS:
- Do not sway your torso back and forth.
- Do not allow your elbows to rise off the bench.
- Maintain good posture with your back straight at all times.
- Do not allow your arms to straighten all the way. Always keep a slight bend in the elbows in order to protect them from injury.
- Keep yourself seated. Do not allow yourself to rise from the seat during the motion.
- You may also perform this exercise with a thumb up position or hammer grip by using a rope handle.

DIFFICULTY -	⊢⊣ �	
♂	STARTING WEIGHT - 40	
♀	STARTING WEIGHT - 20	

ONE ARM CABLE PREACHER CURL

MAJOR MUSCLES IN USE:
Biceps Brachii, Brachialis

STARTING POSITION:
- Sit at a preacher bench so that the bottom portion of your chest is level with and pushed in tightly against the top of the bench.
- Take an underhand grip on a single handle that is attached to the low pulley of the pulley machine. Position your hand so that it is below, but in line with your shoulder. The non-exercising arm can be placed across the top of the bench.

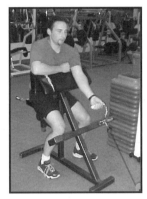

START

EXERCISE MOVEMENT:
- While keeping your torso stationary, begin by lifting the handle along a semicircular path towards your chin.
- Finish with your forearm perpendicular to the floor and the handle at mid-face level.
- Lower the weight back along the same path that you lifted it but stop just before your arm straightens. Repeat for the necessary number of repetitions.

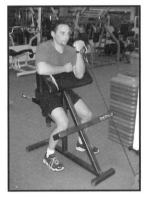

FINISH

EXERCISE TECHNIQUE POINTS:
- Do not sway your torso back and forth.
- Do not allow your elbow to rise off the bench or move from side to side.
- Maintain good posture with your back straight at all times.
- Do not allow your arm to straighten all the way. Always keep a slight bend in the elbow in order to protect it from injury.
- Keep yourself seated. Do not rise from the seat during the exercise.
- You may also perform this exercise with a thumb up position or hammer grip by using one side of a rope handle.

DIFFICULTY - ⊢ ⊢	
♂	STARTING WEIGHT - 15
♀	STARTING WEIGHT - 10

CONCENTRATION CURL

MAJOR MUSCLES IN USE:
Biceps Brachii, Brachialis

STARTING POSITION:
- Sit at the end of a bench and position your feet far apart.
- Grasp a dumbbell with one hand and place your arm so that the back of your elbow is pressed firmly into the middle of the inside of your thigh.
- The palm of your hand should be facing away from your thigh and your arm should be hanging straight down.
- Brace your other arm on your opposite knee.

EXERCISE MOVEMENT:
- While keeping your upper arm and torso stationary, begin by bending the elbow and lifting the dumbbells upward in a semicircular arc following the natural curve of your arm movement.
- At midpoint in the motion, your elbows should be bent at 90° with your forearm parallel to the floor and your upper arm perpendicular to the floor.
- Finish with the dumbbell in front of your shoulder with your upper arm remaining perpendicular to the floor and the back of your hand facing away from your shoulder.
- Return the weight to the starting position while not allowing your torso to move.
- Before you start another repetition, your arm should once again be straight.

EXERCISE TECHNIQUE POINTS:
- Do not sway your torso back and forth.
- Do not allow your elbow to move up or down as you raise and lower the weight.
- Make sure your arm is completely straight before starting another repetition.
- You may also perform this exercise with a thumb up position or hammer grip.

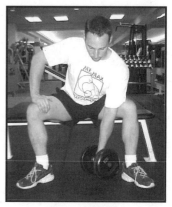

START

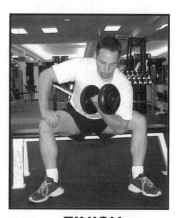

FINISH

DIFFICULTY -	H H	
♂	STARTING WEIGHT - 15	
♀	STARTING WEIGHT - 10	

BICEPS EXERCISES

CABLE CONCENTRATION CURL

MAJOR MUSCLES IN USE:
Biceps Brachii, Brachialis

STARTING POSITION:
- Position the end of an exercise bench in front of the low pulley of a pulley machine. Sit at the end of the bench and position your feet far apart.
- Grasp a single handle attached to the low pulley of a pulley machine with one hand and place your arm so that the back of your elbow is pressed firmly into the middle of the inside of your thigh.
- The palm of your hand should be facing away from your thigh and your arm should be hanging straight down.
- Place your other hand on your opposite knee.

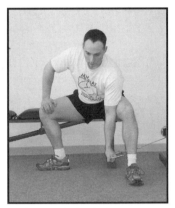

START

EXERCISE MOVEMENT:
- While keeping your upper arm and torso stationary, begin by bending the elbow and lifting the handle upward in a semicircular arc following the natural curve of your arm movement.
- At midpoint in the motion, your elbows should be bent at 90° with your forearm parallel to the floor and your upper arm perpendicular to the floor.
- Finish with the dumbbell in front of your shoulder with your upper arm remaining perpendicular to the floor and the back of your hand facing away from your shoulder.
- Return the handle to the starting position while not allowing your torso to move.
- Before you start another repetition, your arm should once again be straight.

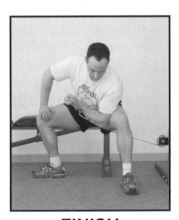

FINISH

EXERCISE TECHNIQUE POINTS:
- Do not sway your torso back and forth.
- Do not allow your elbow to move up or down as you raise and lower the weight.
- Make sure your arm is completely straight before starting another repetition.
- You may also perform this motion with one end of a rope handle.

DIFFICULTY -	⊢⊣ ⊢⊣	
♂	STARTING WEIGHT - 15	
♀	STARTING WEIGHT - 10	

BARBELL CONCENTRATION CURL

MAJOR MUSCLES IN USE:
Biceps Brachii, Brachialis

STARTING POSITION:
- Stand with feet wider than shoulder width apart and your knees slightly bent.
- Bend over at the waist with your hips and buttocks pushed out, forming a slight curve in your lower back. Your upper back should be flat. Your upper back will flatten if you keep your chest up.
- Grasp the bar with a chest-width, underhand grip. Keep the bar close to your legs and brace your elbows in front of your knees. Your abdominal muscles should be tensed. Your upper back should be parallel to the floor.

EXERCISE MOVEMENT:
- While keeping your upper arms stationary, begin by allowing your elbows to bend as you lift the weight in a semicircular motion.
- At the midpoint of the movement, your arms should be bent with your forearms parallel to the floor and your upper arms perpendicular to the floor.
- Finish with the barbell close to shoulder level. Your upper arms should remain perpendicular to the floor.
- Return the weight to the starting position while not allowing your elbows to move backwards.
- Before you start another repetition, your arms should be straight.

EXERCISE TECHNIQUE POINTS:
- Do not sway your torso back and forth.
- Brace your upper arms and elbows against your legs.
- Do not allow your elbows to move forwards as you lift the weight up.
- Maintain good posture with your back straight at all times.
- Do not bend your knees or "jump" the weight up to complete a repetition.

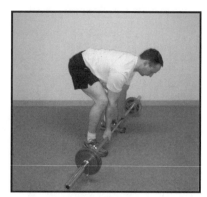

START

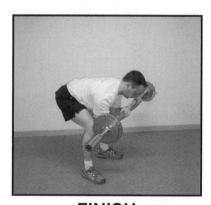

FINISH

DIFFICULTY - ⊢	
♂	STARTING WEIGHT - 40
♀	STARTING WEIGHT - 20

BODY DRAG CURL

MAJOR MUSCLES IN USE:
Biceps Brachii, Brachialis

STARTING POSITION:
- Stand with knees slightly bent and feet about shoulder width apart.
- Grasp the barbell with an underhand grip with your hands positioned about shoulder width apart.
- Arms should hang straight down at your sides with the bar resting on your upper thighs.

EXERCISE MOVEMENT:
- Keeping the bar close to your body, bend your elbows by allowing them to move back as you lift the weight up. The bar should follow the contours of your body.
- Finish with the barbell at about chest level and your elbows fully bent.
- Return the weight to the starting position while not allowing the bar to move away from your body.
- Before you start another repetition, your arms should once again be straight.

EXERCISE TECHNIQUE POINTS:
- Do not sway your torso back and forth.
- Maintain good posture with your back straight at all times.
- Do not bend your knees or "jump" the weight up to complete a repetition.

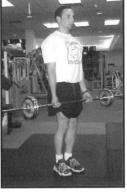

START

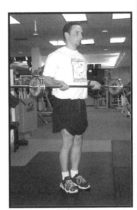

MIDDLE

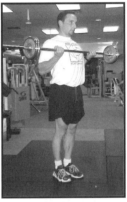

FINISH

DIFFICULTY -	H	H	H
♂ STARTING WEIGHT - 45			
♀ STARTING WEIGHT - 25			

BICEPS EXERCISES

SPIDER CURL

MAJOR MUSCLES IN USE:
Biceps Brachii, Brachialis

STARTING POSITION:
- Position yourself backwards and facing the floor on an inclining bench set at about 40° to the floor so that your chest is resting against the backrest and your legs are placed on either side of the bench.
- Take a dumbbell in each hand and let your arms hang down on either side of the bench. Position your upper body higher on the backrest so that your head is above the top portion of the bench.
- Position your palms facing forward.

EXERCISE MOVEMENT:
- While keeping your upper arms stationary, begin by bending your arms at the elbows and lifting the dumbbells upwards following the natural curve of your arm movement.
- At midpoint in the motion, your elbows should be bent at 90° with your forearms parallel to the floor and your upper arms perpendicular to the floor.
- Finish with the dumbbells in front of your shoulders with your upper arms remaining perpendicular to the floor and the backs of your hands facing directly forward.
- Return the weight to the starting position while not allowing your elbows to move backwards.
- Before you start another repetition, your arms should once again be straight.

EXERCISE TECHNIQUE POINTS:
- Do not allow your elbows to move backwards or forwards as you lift the weight.
- You may also perform this exercise with a thumb up position or hammer grip.

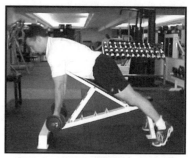

START

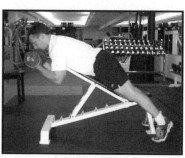

FINISH

DIFFICULTY -	H H H
♂ STARTING WEIGHT - 15	
♀ STARTING WEIGHT - 8	

CLOSE GRIP CHINS

MAJOR MUSCLES IN USE:

Latissimus Dorsi, Biceps Brachii, Brachialis, Posterior Deltoid

STARTING POSITION:

- Grasp the chin-up bar using an underhand grip and place your hands a little closer than shoulder width apart.
- While hanging from the bar with your arms straight, stabilize your shoulders by tensing the shoulder and back muscles.
- Keep your feet off the floor as you do the exercise.

EXERCISE MOVEMENT:

- Begin by using your arms' strength to pull yourself up. As you pull yourself up, try to stay as vertical as possible to allow your biceps muscles to do most of the lifting.
- As you approach the chin-up bar, you will most likely have to lean back slightly in order to clear the bar.
- Try to touch your upper chest to the bar. If this is not possible, you should be able to lift yourself high enough so that your chin is level with the bar.
- Lower yourself back to the starting position so that your arms are fully extended.

EXERCISE TECHNIQUE POINTS:

- Make sure you pull yourself up smoothly without any jerking or kicking movements.
- Make sure your arms are fully extended at the bottom. If you cannot pull yourself up from a fully extended position or you cannot pull yourself high enough, you are not strong enough yet to do this exercise or you may need the help of a spotter.

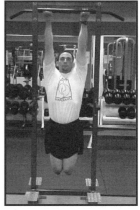

START

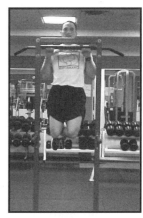

FINISH

DIFFICULTY - H H		
♂	STARTING WEIGHT - no weight	
♀	STARTING WEIGHT - no weight	

BICEPS EXERCISES

HIGH PULLEY DOUBLE BICEPS CURLS

MAJOR MUSCLES IN USE:
Biceps Brachii, Brachialis

STARTING POSITION:
- This exercise requires a special cable cross-over machine or an exercise set-up of two pulldown machines facing each other.
- Grasp each handle from the high pulley with the hand that is closest to it and position yourself in the middle of the machine. Stand straight with feet about shoulder width apart.
- Your arms should be straight with your palms facing up so that your body takes on the position of a very shallow "Y".

EXERCISE MOVEMENT:
- While keeping your upper arms stationary and your elbows pointing away from your body and to the side, begin the movement by bringing the handles towards your ears.
- At the end point in the movement, each handle should be at ear level and a few inches away from your head.
- Finish the exercise by returning the handles back to the starting position along the same line that you used to pull the handles together.

EXERCISE TECHNIQUE POINTS:
- Remember to stand straight.
- Keep your elbows pointing directly out to the sides and your upper arms stationary.
- Do not twist the handles during any part of the movement.
- You may also perform this exercise with a thumb up position or hammer grip.

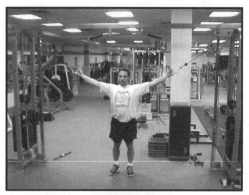

START

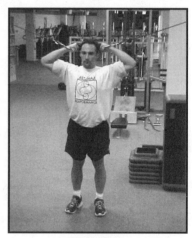

FINISH

DIFFICULTY -	H H H		
♂	STARTING WEIGHT - 20		
♀	STARTING WEIGHT - 10		

BICEPS EXERCISES

LOW PULLEY DOUBLE BICEPS CURLS

MAJOR MUSCLES IN USE:
Biceps Brachii, Brachialis

STARTING POSITION:
- This exercise requires a special cable cross-over machine or an exercise set-up of two pulldown machines facing each other.
- Grasp each single handle from the low pulley with the corresponding closest hand and position yourself in the middle of the machine(s). Stand straight with feet about shoulder width apart.
- Your arms should be straight, palms facing up, arms are directly out to the sides, and your hands level with your hips.

EXERCISE MOVEMENT:
- While keeping your upper arms stationary and your arms pointing outwards and to the sides, begin the movement by bringing the handles towards your shoulders.
- At the end point in the movement, the handles should be at shoulder level and only a few inches away from your shoulders.
- Finish the exercise by returning the handles back to the starting position along the same line that you used to raise them.

EXERCISE TECHNIQUE POINTS:
- Remember to stand up straight.
- Remember to keep your elbows pointing directly out to the sides and your upper arms stationary.
- Do not twist the handles during any part of the movement.
- You may also perform this exercise with a thumb up position or hammer grip.

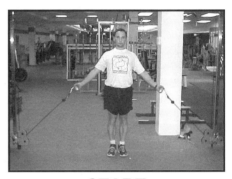

START

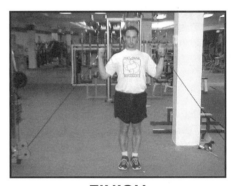

FINISH

DIFFICULTY -	⊢⊢ ⊢⊢ ⊢⊢		
♂	STARTING WEIGHT - 20
♀	STARTING WEIGHT - 10

BICEPS EXERCISES 281

VERTICAL CABLE CURLS

MAJOR MUSCLES IN USE:
Biceps Brachii, Brachialis

STARTING POSITION:
- Kneeling in front of a pulley machine, take an underhand grip with hands about shoulder width apart on a bar attached to the high pulley of a cable machine.
- Allow your arms to straighten so that the bar is directly above your head.
- Keep your chest up and your back straight and tense your shoulder muscles to help stabilize your arms.

EXERCISE MOVEMENT:
- While keeping your upper arms stationary, begin by bending your arms at the elbows and pull the bar down following the natural arc of your arm movement.
- Finish with the bar behind your head at the base of your skull. Your upper arms should remain almost vertical and the palms of your hands should face downwards.
- Return the bar to the starting position while not allowing your elbows to move.
- Before you start another repetition, your arms should be straight.

EXERCISE TECHNIQUE POINTS:
- Do not sway your torso back and forth.
- Do not allow your elbows to move backwards or forwards as you pull the weight down.
- Maintain good posture with your back straight at all times.
- You may also perform this exercise with a thumb down position or hammer grip using a rope handle.

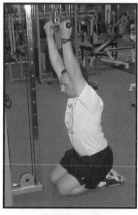

START

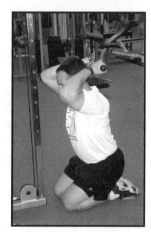

FINISHED

DIFFICULTY -	H	H	H
♂ STARTING WEIGHT - 40			
♀ STARTING WEIGHT - 20			

BICEPS EXERCISES

LYING VERTICAL CABLE CURLS

MAJOR MUSCLES IN USE:
Biceps Brachii, Brachialis

STARTING POSITION:
- Take an under handgrip with hands about shoulder width apart on a bar attached to the high pulley of a cable machine.
- While hanging onto the bar, lie on your back on a flat bench positioned so that the end of the bench is about 2 feet in front of the pulley machine.
- Allow your arms to straighten so that the bar is directly above your head.
- Keep your chest up and your back straight and tense your shoulder muscles to help stabilize your arms.

EXERCISE MOVEMENT:
- While keeping your upper arms stationary, begin by bending your arms at the elbows and pull the bar downwards.
- At midpoint in the motion, your elbows should be bent at 90° with your forearms parallel to the floor and your upper arms almost perpendicular to the floor.
- Finish with the bar at the top of your head. Your upper arms should remain almost vertical and the palms of your hands should face towards your head.
- Return the bar to the starting position while not allowing your elbows to move.
- Before starting another repetition, make sure your arms are straight.

EXERCISE TECHNIQUE POINTS:
- Do not allow your elbows to move backwards, forwards, or outwards as you pull the weight down.
- Maintain good posture by keeping your back straight and not arching your lower back.
- You may also perform this exercise with a thumb down position or hammer grip using a rope handle.

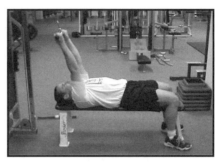

START

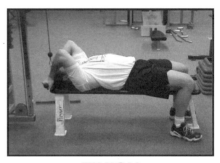

FINISH

DIFFICULTY -	⊢	⊢	⊢
♂ STARTING WEIGHT - 40			
♀ STARTING WEIGHT - 20			

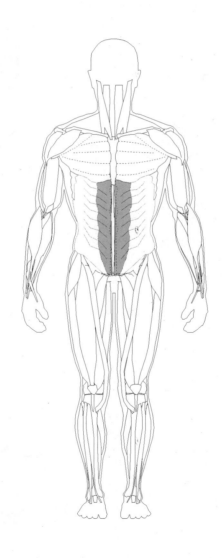

FULL INCLINE CRUNCH

MAJOR MUSCLES IN USE:
Rectus Abdominus, External Oblique, Rectus Femoris

STARTING POSITION:
- Lying on an abdominal board with your head lower than your feet, hook your feet into the end pads or available loops.
- Your knees should be bent at approximately 90°.
- Hands can be either crossed across the upper chest or placed at the ears.

EXERCISE MOVEMENT:
- Begin the movement by curling your torso upwards, allowing your shoulders to rise off the bench first followed by your shoulder blades, then by your middle back, and finally by your lower back.
- You should finish the movement with your torso perpendicular to the floor.
- Return to the starting position by uncurling your torso in the reverse order (lower back should touch the bench first, then middle back, shoulder blades, and finally shoulders).

EXERCISE TECHNIQUE POINTS:
- Do not bounce your torso off the bench in order to complete the necessary repetitions.
- Do not allow your hips to lift off the bench in order to help you pull yourself to the finish position.
- You should not allow your pelvis to tilt forward resulting in an arching of your lower back during the beginning of the movement.
- Your back should round as you go from the starting position to the final position.
- You may also make it more challenging by holding a weight to your chest or behind your head.

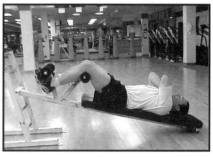

START

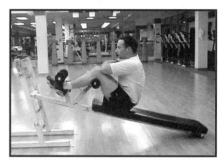

FINISH

DIFFICULTY -	H	
♂	STARTING LEVEL - Flat	
♀	STARTING LEVEL - Flat	

ABDOMINAL EXERCISES

ROMAN CHAIR SIT-UP

MAJOR MUSCLES IN USE:
Rectus Abdominus, External Oblique, Rectus Femoris

STARTING POSITION:
- Sit on a roman chair bench, hyperextension bench, or at the end of a flat bench with your feet securely fastened by either a leg attachment or by someone you trust completely holding your feet.
- Place your feet under the leg pads of the bench.
- Hands can be crossed across the upper chest or placed beside the ears.

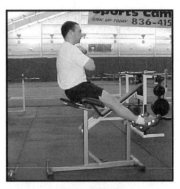

START

EXERCISE MOVEMENT:
- Begin the movement by lowering yourself backwards so that you finish with your body even with or just below the level of the bench.
- Raise yourself back to the starting position by curling your torso upwards allowing your upper back to round as you rise up.
- You should finish the movement with your torso perpendicular to the floor.

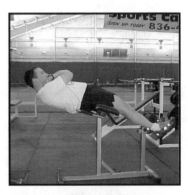

FINISH

EXERCISE TECHNIQUE POINTS:
- Do not lower yourself much below the level of the bench as this could place added and undesirable strain on your lower back.
- Make sure that your feet are fastened very securely either by the leg hold attachments or the person holding your feet.
- You should not allow your pelvis to tilt forward at any point in the movement.
- You may also make it more challenging by holding a weight to your chest or behind your head.

DIFFICULTY -	H	H	H
♂ STARTING LEVEL - Body			
♀ STARTING LEVEL - Body			

WEIGHT RESISTED INCLINE CRUNCH

MAJOR MUSCLES IN USE:
Rectus Abdominus, External Oblique, Rectus Femoris

STARTING POSITION:
- Lying on an incline board with your head lower than your feet, hook your feet into the end pads or available loops.
- Hold onto a dumbbell or barbell plate so that it rests on your upper chest. Generally, the most comfortable way to hang onto the weight is to cross your arms over top so that you are holding on to the sides of the weight. To make the exercise more challenging, place the dumbbell behind your upper neck instead of your chest.

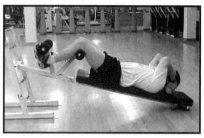

START

EXERCISE MOVEMENT:
- Begin the movement by curling your torso upwards, first raising your shoulders off the incline bench, followed by your shoulder blades, middle back, and finally by your lower back.
- You should finish the movement with your torso perpendicular to the floor.
- Return to the starting position by uncurling your torso in the reverse order (lower back should touch first, then middle back, shoulder blades, and finally shoulders).

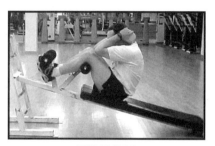

FINISH

EXERCISE TECHNIQUE POINTS:
- Do not bounce your torso off the bench in order to complete the necessary repetitions.
- Do not allow your hips to lift off the bench in order to help you pull yourself up.
- You should not allow your pelvis to tilt forward while arching your lower back at the beginning of the movement.

DIFFICULTY -	⊢⊣ ⊢⊣	
♂	STARTING LEVEL - Flat	
♀	STARTING LEVEL - Flat	

CABLE CRUNCH

MAJOR MUSCLES IN USE:
Rectus Abdominus, External Oblique

STARTING POSITION:
- Kneeling on the floor in front of a pulldown machine, grasp a rope handle attached to the high pulley and position your hands beside your ears or just in front of your forehead. Arch your back by holding your chest high.
- Sit on the backs of your heels and remain there throughout the whole motion.

EXERCISE MOVEMENT:
- Begin the movement by first bringing your shoulders downwards so that you are rounding your upper back, but not bending at the waist. Try to think about bringing your ribcage down towards your pelvis.
- You should finish the movement with your elbows near your thighs and your back rounded as much as possible.
- Return to the starting position by reversing the order used when you pulled down on the cable. You should finish with your back arched and your chest held high again.

EXERCISE TECHNIQUE POINTS:
- Do not lean forward by bending at the waist in order to move the weight.
- Do not allow your hands to move from your ears or your forehead when performing the exercise.
- Make sure to arch your back up and raise your chest as high as possible (while you are sitting on your heels) at the beginning of each repetition.

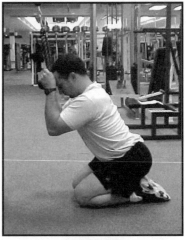

START

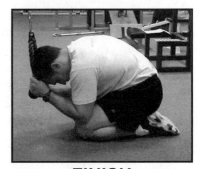

FINISH

DIFFICULTY -	⊢ ⊢ ⊢ ⊦
♂ STARTING WEIGHT - 50	
♀ STARTING WEIGHT - 30	

ABDOMINAL EXERCISES

FLOOR CRUNCH

MAJOR MUSCLES IN USE:
Rectus Abdominus, External Oblique

STARTING POSITION:
- Lie on the floor with your knees bent at 90° and feet flat on the floor. If you wish, you may choose to support your feet on a chair or a bench.
- Hands can be crossed on your upper chest, placed beside your ears, or placed flat against your thighs.

EXERCISE MOVEMENT:
- Begin the movement by curling your torso upwards off the floor towards your knees. Lead with your shoulders, your shoulder blades, middle back, and if you are particularly strong, your lower back.
- You should finish the movement with your shoulders as high off the ground as possible.
- Return to the starting position by reversing the order (lower back should touch first, then middle back, shoulder blades, and finally the shoulders).

EXERCISE TECHNIQUE POINTS:
- Do not bounce your torso off the floor in order to complete the necessary repetitions.
- Make sure that you raise your shoulders as high as possible.
- Be very careful that you do not excessively bend the neck in order to complete your repetitions.
- The torso should curl or roll up so that your back rounds as you go from the starting position to the finish position.

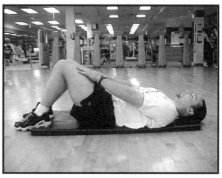

START

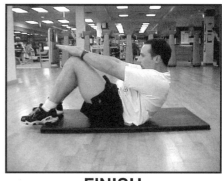

FINISH

DIFFICULTY -	⊢|
♂	STARTING LEVEL - Hands Out
♀	STARTING LEVEL - Hands Out

BALL CRUNCH

MAJOR MUSCLES IN USE:
Rectus Abdominus, External Oblique

STARTING POSITION:
- Sit on the edge of an exercise ball with your legs bent slightly more than 90° and your feet wider than shoulder width.
- Hands can be crossed across the upper chest, placed beside the ears, or placed flat against the thighs.

EXERCISE MOVEMENT:
- Begin the movement by leaning back while allowing the ball to roll slightly forward.
- You should finish the movement with your back in full contact with the ball.
- Return to the starting position by curling your torso up by first raising your shoulders, then your shoulder blades, then your middle back, and finally your lower back.

EXERCISE TECHNIQUE POINTS:
- Do not bounce your torso off the ball in order to complete the necessary repetitions.
- Make sure that you round your upper back as you curl up.
- Keep your feet wider apart than shoulder width to help you balance.
- You may also make it more challenging by holding a weight to your chest or behind your head.

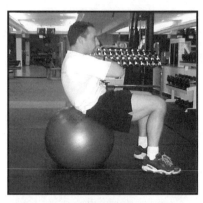

START

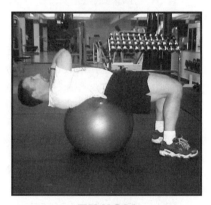

FINISH

DIFFICULTY -	⊢ ⊢ ⊢	
♂	STARTING LEVEL	- no weight
♀	STARTING LEVEL	- no weight

BALL CABLE CRUNCH

MAJOR MUSCLES IN USE:
Rectus Abdominus, External Oblique

STARTING POSITION:
- Place an exercise ball in front of a low pulley of a pulley machine. Attach a rope handle to the cable.
- Sit on the edge of an exercise ball with your back facing the machine. Your legs should be bent slightly more than 90° and your feet wider than shoulder width.
- Lean back allowing the ball to roll slightly forward and grasp a rope handle. Position your hands on either side of your neck at the level of your upper chest.

EXERCISE MOVEMENT:
- Begin the movement by curling your torso up by first raising your shoulders, then your shoulder blades, then your middle back, and finally your lower back.
- Once you have reached a sitting position, return to the starting position by reversing the movement along the same path.

EXERCISE TECHNIQUE POINTS:
- Do not bounce your torso off the ball in order to complete the necessary repetitions.
- Make sure that you round your upper back as you curl up.
- Keep your feet wider apart than shoulder width to help you balance.
- If you find yourself being pulled back towards the machine, try repositioning your body by lowering your hips on the ball.

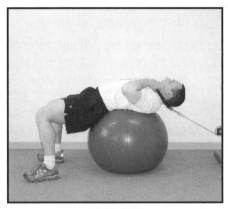

START

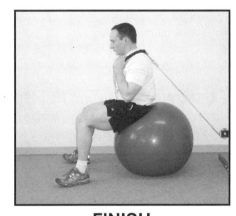

FINISH

DIFFICULTY -	⊢⊣ ⊢⊣ ⊢	
♂	STARTING LEVEL - 20	
♀	STARTING LEVEL - 10	

BALL PIKES

MAJOR MUSCLES IN USE:
Rectus Abdominus, External Oblique, Rectus Femoris

STARTING POSITION:
- Place both your feet and your shins on an exercise ball and fully extend your legs so that your body is in a straight line.
- You should now be positioned in a push-up position with your arms locked, your hands placed wider than shoulder width apart, and the tops of your feet on top of the ball.

EXERCISE MOVEMENT:
- While keeping your upper torso stationary and your legs straight, raise your hips upwards by allowing the ball to roll forward towards your torso.
- Focus on bringing the ball towards your hands as much as possible so that the pelvis tilts forward.
- Return the ball back to the starting position so that your body is straight.

EXERCISE TECHNIQUE POINTS:
- Try not to let the ball move from side to side while doing the exercise.
- Make sure that your upper thighs are in a straight line with your torso as you begin the exercise and that you get a good tilt in the pelvis at the end.
- Try to keep your abdominal muscles as tight as possible.
- Always try to keep your hips as high as possible throughout the movement.
- If you find it difficult to bring the ball forward at the end of the movement try stretching your hamstrings before performing the exercise.

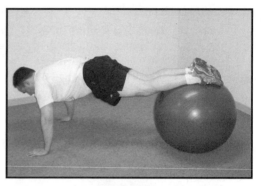

START

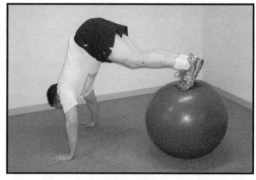

FINISH

DIFFICULTY -	H H H H H
♂	STARTING LEVEL - no weight
♀	STARTING LEVEL - no weight

BALL KNEE TUCKS

MAJOR MUSCLES IN USE:
Rectus Abdominus, External Oblique, Rectus Femoris

STARTING POSITION:
- Place both your feet and your shins on an exercise ball and fully extend your legs so that your body is in a straight line.
- You should now be positioned in a push-up position with your arms locked, your hands placed wider than shoulder width apart, and your feet on top of the ball.

EXERCISE MOVEMENT:
- While keeping your upper torso stationary, pull the ball towards your torso by bending your legs at the knees.
- Focus on bringing the knees forward and into your chest as much as possible so that the pelvis tilts forward.
- Return the ball back to the starting position so that your body is straight.

EXERCISE TECHNIQUE POINTS:
- Try not to let the ball move from side to side while doing the exercise.
- Make sure that your upper thighs are in a straight line with your torso as you begin the exercise and that you get a good tilt in the pelvis at the end.
- Try to keep your abdominal muscles as tight as possible.

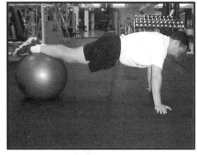
START

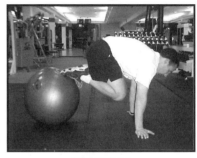
FINISH

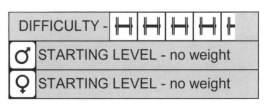

DIFFICULTY -	H H H H H
♂	STARTING LEVEL - no weight
♀	STARTING LEVEL - no weight

BALL REVERSE CRUNCH

MAJOR MUSCLES IN USE:
Rectus Abdominus, External Oblique

STARTING POSITION:
- Lie on the floor with your legs bent at 90°, thighs perpendicular and calves parallel to the floor. Place an exercise ball between your feet and hold it in position.
- Arms should be extended straight down beside your body so that your hands are lower than your hips.

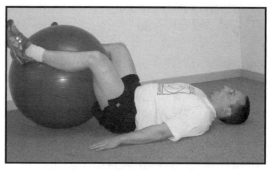

START

EXERCISE MOVEMENT:
- Begin the movement by tightening your abdominal muscles and raising your hips off the floor so that your hips curve upwards as the ball rises.
- You should finish the movement with your hips raised off the ground as high as possible and the ball directly above you.
- Return to the starting position by reversing the motion and lowering the ball to the floor.

EXERCISE TECHNIQUE POINTS:
- Do not bounce your hips and the ball off the floor in order to complete the necessary repetitions.
- Let your pelvis tilt forward at the top portion of the movement.
- The torso should curl up as you go from the start to finish positions.
- Make sure you have the ball in the proper position before starting the movement.

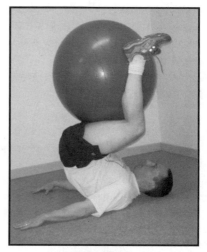

FINISH

DIFFICULTY -	H	H	H
♂ STARTING LEVEL - knees close			
♀ STARTING LEVEL - knees close			

ABDOMINAL EXERCISES

REVERSE CRUNCH

MAJOR MUSCLES IN USE:
Rectus Abdominus, External Oblique

STARTING POSITION:
- Lie on the floor with your legs bent at 90°, thighs perpendicular and calves parallel to the floor. Cross your ankles to help keep your legs together.
- Arms should be extended straight down beside your body so that your hands are lower than your hips.

EXERCISE MOVEMENT:
- Begin the movement by tightening your abdominal muscles and raising your hips off the floor so that your hips curve upwards.
- You should finish the movement with your hips raised off the ground as high as possible. If you find this movement too difficult to perform properly, you can try instead to bring the knees in closer to your chest.
- Return to the starting position by reversing the motion.

EXERCISE TECHNIQUE POINTS:
- Do not bounce your hips off the floor in order to complete the necessary repetitions.
- Let your pelvis tilt forward at the top portion of the movement.
- The torso should curl up as you go from the start to finish positions.

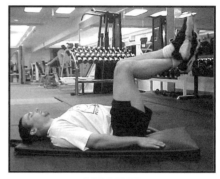

START

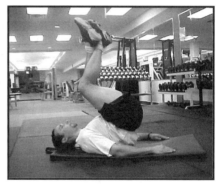

FINISH

DIFFICULTY -	⊢⊣	⊢⊣	
♂	STARTING LEVEL - knees close		
♀	STARTING LEVEL - knees close		

LEG RAISE

MAJOR MUSCLES IN USE:
Rectus Abdominus, External Oblique

STARTING POSITION:
- Lie flat on the floor on your back. Position your hands underneath your hips.
- Raise your feet so that they are approximately 6 inches off the ground and bend your knees slightly.

EXERCISE MOVEMENT:
- Begin the movement by raising your legs and feet away from the following an upwards arc.
- You should finish the movement with your thighs at least perpendicular to the floor. If you find this too difficult you can pull the knees in closer to the chest.
- Return to the starting position by reversing the movement.

EXERCISE TECHNIQUE POINTS:
- Do not allow your body to rock back and forth as you perform your repetitions.
- Do not allow your knees to carry over your head as this can put added strain on the back.
- The torso should curl or roll up and the back will round as you go from the starting position to the finish position.
- If you find this motion too difficult you may start with your knees bent at a 90° angle. The straighter your legs are, the more difficult the exercise.
- You may also make it more challenging by holding a dumbbell between your feet or by using ankle weights.

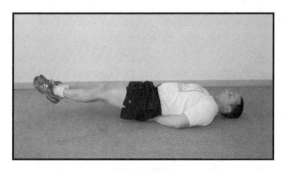

START

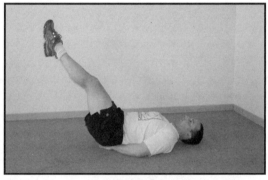

FINISH

DIFFICULTY -	H
♂	STARTING LEVEL - no weight
♀	STARTING LEVEL - no weight

ABDOMINAL BRIDGING

MAJOR MUSCLES IN USE:
Rectus Abdominus, External Oblique

STARTING POSITION:
- Place your feet on the floor with your legs fully extended so that your body is in a straight line.
- Place your forearms on the floor so that your upper body is resting on your elbows.
- No other part of your body other than your feet and your forearms should touch the floor.

EXERCISE MOVEMENT:
- There is no movement to this exercise. The challenge for the abdominal muscles is to hold the position as long as possible.

EXERCISE TECHNIQUE POINTS:
- Make sure you keep your body perfectly straight.
- Try to keep your abdominal muscles and lower back muscles as tight as possible.
- If you find your elbows are uncomfortable try performing the exercise on a mat or place your arms on a pillow.
- To add extra resistance have a partner place a light weight on your hips.

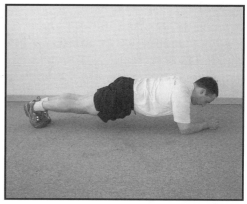

START AND FINISH

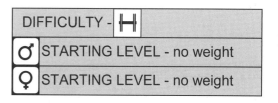

DIFFICULTY - ⊦⊣		
♂	STARTING LEVEL - no weight	
♀	STARTING LEVEL - no weight	

BALL BRIDGING

MAJOR MUSCLES IN USE:
Rectus Abdominus, External Oblique

STARTING POSITION:
- Place both your feet on top of an exercise ball and fully extend your legs so that your body is in a straight line.
- You should now be positioned in a push-up position with your arms locked, your hands placed wider than shoulder width apart, and your feet on top of the ball.

EXERCISE MOVEMENT:
- There is no movement to this exercise. The challenge for the abdominal muscles is to hold the position as long as possible.

EXERCISE TECHNIQUE POINTS:
- Make sure you keep your body perfectly straight.
- Try to keep your abdominal muscles and lower back muscles as tight as possible.
- If you find your elbows are uncomfortable try performing the exercise on a mat or place your arms on a pillow.
- To add extra resistance have a partner place a light weight on your hips.

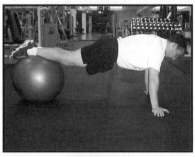
START

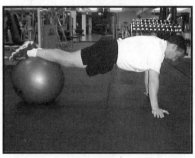
FINISH

DIFFICULTY - ⊢⊣ ⊢⊣ ⊢		
♂	STARTING LEVEL – no weight	
♀	STARTING LEVEL – no weight	

BALL ROLL-OUTS

MAJOR MUSCLES IN USE:
Rectus Abdominus, External Oblique

STARTING POSITION:
- Place both your feet shoulder width apart on the floor and support your upper body with your forearms on the side closest to you of an exercise ball.

EXERCISE MOVEMENT:
- While keeping your upper torso stationary, extend your arms allowing the ball to roll away from your body.
- Focus on keeping your body as straight as possible by tensing your abdominal and lower back exercises.
- Return the ball back to the starting position so that your elbows are once again supporting your upper body.

EXERCISE TECHNIQUE POINTS:
- Try not to let the ball move from side to side while doing the exercise.
- Make sure that your upper thighs are in a straight line with your hips and torso as you begin the exercise and that you extend your arms as far as possible.
- Try to keep your abdominal and lower back muscles as tight as possible.
- This exercise is very challenging on the abdominal muscles thereby giving it a difficulty rating of 5.

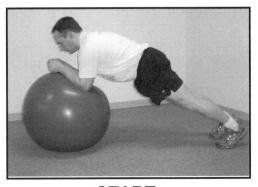

START

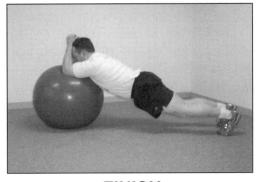

FINISH

DIFFICULTY -	H	H	H	H	H
♂ STARTING LEVEL - N/A					
♀ STARTING LEVEL - N/A					

INCLINE LEG RAISE

MAJOR MUSCLES IN USE:
Rectus Abdominus, External Oblique

STARTING POSITION:
- Lie on an abdominal board with your head higher than your feet. Steady your upper body by grabbing onto the end pads or available loops.
- Your knees should be bent at a minimum angle of 90°. Cross your feet in order to keep your legs together during the exercise.

EXERCISE MOVEMENT:
- Begin the movement by raising your hips up off the incline bench so that your hips follow an upwards arc.
- You should finish the movement with your thighs at least perpendicular to the floor. If you find this too difficult you can pull the knees in closer to the chest.
- Return to the starting position by reversing the movement.

EXERCISE TECHNIQUE POINTS:
- Do not bounce your hips off the bench in order to complete the necessary repetitions.
- Do not allow your knees to carry over your head as this can put added strain on the back.
- Allow your pelvis to tilt forward and try to keep your knees as far away from your chest as possible.
- The torso should curl or roll up and the back will round as you go from the starting position to the finish position.

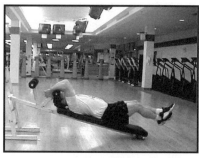

START

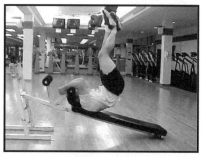

FINISH

DIFFICULTY -	H	H	H
♂ STARTING LEVEL - Flat			
♀ STARTING LEVEL - Flat			

ABDOMINAL EXERCISES 300

SEATED LEG RAISE or "V's"

MAJOR MUSCLES IN USE:
Rectus Abdominus, External Oblique, Rectus Femoris

STARTING POSITION:
- Sit at the edge of an exercise bench and lean back far enough so that you are balanced when you take your feet off the ground.
- Hang onto the exercise bench or place your hands behind you to provide extra stability.
- Your body should be as straight as possible and at a slight angle to the floor.

EXERCISE MOVEMENT:
- Begin the movement by raising your legs, allowing your pelvis to tilt back as your legs rise. If you find this difficult, you can bend your knees and pull your legs in towards your body.
- You should finish the movement with your feet held as high as possible.
- Return to the starting position by reversing the motion.

EXERCISE TECHNIQUE POINTS:
- Make sure your upper thighs are in a straight line with your torso when you begin and that your pelvis tilts at the end of the movement.
- Balance yourself by adjusting how far back you lean throughout the exercise movement.
- Do not continue to do the movement if you find it uncomfortable on your hips or too difficult to keep your balance.

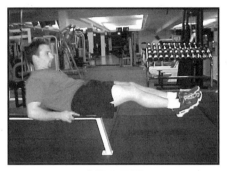

START

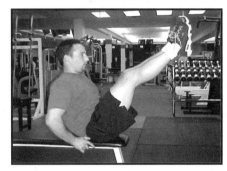

FINISH

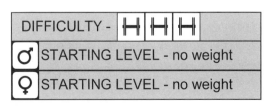

DIFFICULTY -	⫫ ⫫ ⫫	
♂	STARTING LEVEL - no weight	
♀	STARTING LEVEL - no weight	

BALL LEG RAISE

MAJOR MUSCLES IN USE:
Rectus Abdominus, External Oblique, Rectus Femoris

STARTING POSITION:
- Sit on an exercise ball and position yourself between the handles of a dipping station.
- Lean back on the ball, using the handles of the station to steady yourself, so that your feet are off the floor but lower than your shoulders.
- Your torso and upper thighs should form a straight line and your ankles crossed to help keep your legs together.

EXERCISE MOVEMENT:
- Begin the movement by raising your legs upwards, allowing your pelvis to tilt back while steadying yourself with the dip bars.
- You should finish the movement with your thighs perpendicular to the floor. If you find this too difficult, you can pull the knees in closer to the chest.
- Return to the starting position by reversing the movement.

EXERCISE TECHNIQUE POINTS:
- Make sure your upper thighs and your torso form a straight line when you begin and that you have a good tilt to the pelvis at the end.
- Try to keep your knees as far away from your chest as possible.

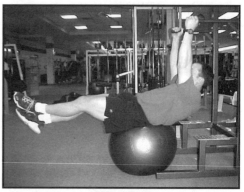

START

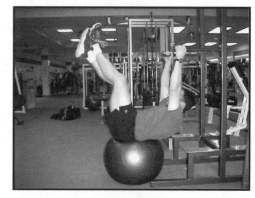

FINISH

DIFFICULTY -	H H H H
♂	STARTING LEVEL - top of ball
♀	STARTING LEVEL - top of ball

HANGING LEG RAISE

MAJOR MUSCLES IN USE:
Rectus Abdominus, External Oblique, Rectus Femoris

STARTING POSITION:
- To perform this exercise you may wish to hang from a chinning bar, support yourself by using dipping bars, or use a special upright leg raise machine.
- Your knees can be bent at an angle of 90° or just slightly bent depending on your abdominal strength. Cross your ankles in order to help keep them together during the exercise.

EXERCISE MOVEMENT:
- Begin the movement by lifting your legs and curling your hips upwards. Your legs and hips should follow a semicircular path upwards.
- You should finish the movement with your knees and feet held as high as possible while your upper body stays perpendicular to the floor. If you find this too difficult, you can pull the knees in closer to the chest.
- Return to the starting position by reversing the movement.

EXERCISE TECHNIQUE POINTS:
- Do not swing your legs in order to complete the necessary repetitions.
- Do not lift your legs with your knees straight.
- Allow your pelvis to tilt forward and try to keep your feet as far away from your body as possible.

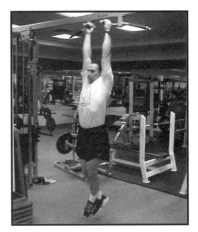

START

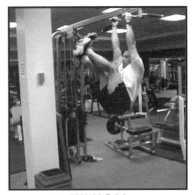

FINISH

DIFFICULTY -	⊢ ⊢ ⊢ ⊢
♂	STARTING LEVEL - knees bent
♀	STARTING LEVEL - knees bent

OBLIQUE EXERCISES

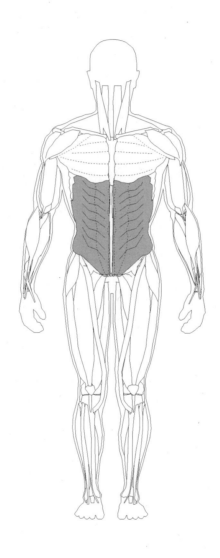

INCLINE TWIST CRUNCH

MAJOR MUSCLES IN USE:
Rectus Abdominus, External Oblique, Rectus Femoris

STARTING POSITION:
- Lie on an abdominal bench with your head lower than your feet. Hook your feet under the end pads or into the available loops.
- Your knees should be bent at approximately 90°.
- Hands can be crossed across the upper chest or placed at the ears.

EXERCISE MOVEMENT:
- Begin the movement by curling upwards and lifting your shoulders off the incline bench followed by your shoulder blades, middle back and finally the lower back.
- As you curl up, rotate your trunk to one side so that one of your elbows is on the outside of your opposite knee when you finish.
- You should finish the movement with your torso perpendicular to the floor.
- Return to the starting position in the reverse order (lower back should touch the bench first, then middle back, shoulder blades, and finally shoulders while you move your trunk back to a neutral position).
- Repeat the motion, twisting your torso this time to the other side.

EXERCISE TECHNIQUE POINTS:
- Do not bounce your torso in order to complete the necessary repetitions.
- Do not allow your hips to lift off the bench in order to pull yourself up.
- You should not allow your pelvis to tilt forward and arch your lower back at the beginning of the movement.
- The torso should curl or roll-up so the back rounds as you go from the starting position to the final position.
- Make sure you rotate your trunk as far to the side as possible as you perform the movement.
- You may also make it more challenging by holding a weight to your chest or behind your head.

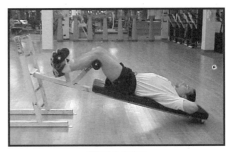

START

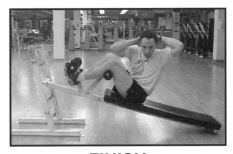

FINISH

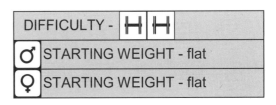

DIFFICULTY -	H	H
♂ STARTING WEIGHT - flat		
♀ STARTING WEIGHT - flat		

OBLIQUE EXERCISES

TWISTING FLOOR CRUNCH

MAJOR MUSCLES IN USE:
Rectus Abdominus, External Oblique

STARTING POSITION:
- Lie on the floor with your knees bent at 90°. You may support your feet on a chair or bench if you wish.
- You may cross your hands across your upper chest, place them beside your ears, or you can hold one arm in front of your body.

EXERCISE MOVEMENT:
- Begin the movement by curling upwards, lifting your shoulders off the floor first, followed by your shoulder blades, your middle back, and then if you are especially strong, your lower back at the same time as you twist your torso to one side.
- You should finish the movement with your shoulders as high off the ground as possible and your torso rotated as far as possible to one side.
- Return to the starting position in the reverse order (lower back should touch the floor first, then middle back, shoulder blades, and finally shoulders).

EXERCISE TECHNIQUE POINTS:
- Do not bounce your torso off the floor in order to complete the necessary repetitions.
- Make sure that your shoulders rise off the ground and twist to one side as far as possible as you perform each repetition.
- Do not bend the neck excessively in order to complete your repetitions.

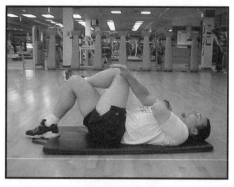

START

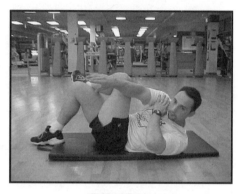

FINISH

DIFFICULTY -	H	
♂	STARTING WEIGHT - no weight	
♀	STARTING WEIGHT - no weight	

OBLIQUE EXERCISES

BICYCLE CRUNCH

MAJOR MUSCLES IN USE:
Rectus Abdominus, External Oblique

STARTING POSITION:
- Lie on the floor with your legs extended and your knees slightly bent. Position your feet about 4 – 6 inches off of the floor.
- You may cross your hands across your upper chest, place them beside your ears, or you can hold them in front of your body.

EXERCISE MOVEMENT:
- Begin the movement by curling upwards, lifting your shoulders off the floor first, followed by your shoulder blades, your middle back, and then if you are especially strong, your lower back at the same time as you twist your torso to one side.
- At the same time as you are performing the above movement, bend the leg on the side to which you are twisting towards and bring the knee in towards the chest.
- You should finish the movement with your trunk rotated as far as possible to one side so that one of your elbows touches the opposite knee when you finish.
- You should finish the movement with your torso and legs suspended off the floor while you balance on your hips.
- Return to the starting position in the reverse order (lower back should touch the floor first, then middle back, shoulder blades, and finally shoulders as you extend the leg back to the starting position).

EXERCISE TECHNIQUE POINTS:
- Do not bounce your torso off the floor in order to complete the necessary repetitions.
- Make sure that your shoulders rise off the ground and twist to one side as far as possible as you perform each repetition.
- Do not bend the neck excessively in order to complete your repetitions.
- Try not to kick your legs to help you lift your torso off the ground.
- Start by lifting your torso first, followed by bending the opposite leg.

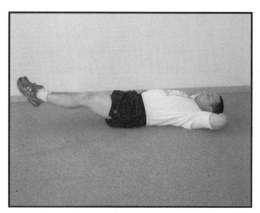

START

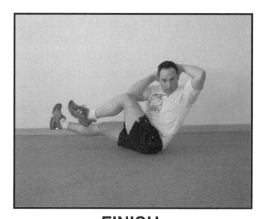

FINISH

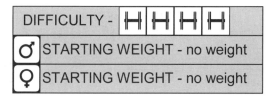

BALL TWIST CRUNCH

MAJOR MUSCLES IN USE:
Rectus Abdominus, External Oblique, Rectus Femoris

STARTING POSITION:
- Sit on the edge of an exercise ball with your legs bent slightly more than 90° and your feet wider than shoulder width.
- Hands can be crossed across the upper chest, placed beside the ears, or held in fron tof the body.
- Lean back while allowing the ball to roll slightly forward. You should finish the movement with your back in full contact with the ball.

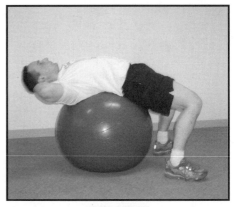

START

EXERCISE MOVEMENT:
- Begin the movement by curling upwards, lifting your shoulders off the ball first, followed by your shoulder blades, your middle back, and then if you are especially strong, your lower back at the same time as you twist your torso to one side.
- As you curl up, rotate your trunk to one side so that you are facing as far as possible to one side.
- You should finish the movement with your torso perpendicular to the floor.
- Return to the starting position in the reverse order (lower back should touch the ball first, then middle back, shoulder blades, and finally shoulders while you move your trunk back to a neutral position).
- Repeat the motion, twisting your torso this time to the other side.

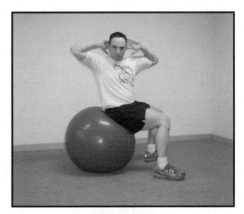

FINISH

EXERCISE TECHNIQUE POINTS:
- Do not bounce your torso off the ball in order to complete the necessary repetitions.
- Make sure that you round your upper back as you curl up.
- Keep your feet wider apart than shoulder width to help you balance.
- Make sure you rotate your trunk as far to the side as possible as you perform the movement.
- You may also make it more challenging by holding a weight to your chest or behind your head.

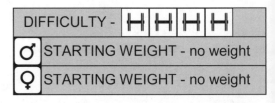

DIFFICULTY - H H H H

♂ STARTING WEIGHT - no weight

♀ STARTING WEIGHT - no weight

TWISTING CABLE CRUNCH

MAJOR MUSCLES IN USE:
Rectus Abdominus, External Oblique

STARTING POSITION:
- Kneel on the floor in front of a cable machine and grasp with both hands a rope handle attached to the high pulley. Position your hands beside your ears or just in front of your forehead. Arch your back by holding your chest high.
- Sit back on your heels with your back arched upwards and your chest held high. Remain seated throughout the whole motion.

EXERCISE MOVEMENT:
- While holding the handle with both hands, begin the movement by bringing your shoulders downwards so that you are rounding your upper back but not bending at the waist. Try to think about bringing your ribcage in and down towards your pelvis.
- As you pull your shoulders down, twist your torso so that one elbow is heading towards the opposite knee.
- You should finish the movement with one of your elbows on the outside of your opposite thigh and with your back curved forward as much as possible.
- Return to the starting position by reversing the motion. You should finish with your back arched and your chest held high again.

EXERCISE TECHNIQUE POINTS:
- Do not lean forward by bending at the waist in order to move the weight.
- You should twist your torso as much as possible as you pull the weight down.
- Make sure you come up as high as you can after each repetition.
- Remember to think about bringing the bottom of your ribcage into your pelvis as you begin the movement.
- Your torso should curl and roll downwards and your back should round as you move from the starting position to the final position.
- Do not allow your hands to move from their initial position.

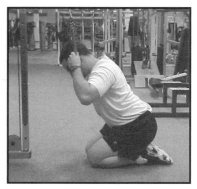

START

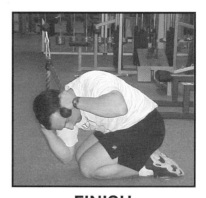

FINISH

DIFFICULTY -	� ⊢⊣⊢⊣⊢⊣⊦
♂ STARTING WEIGHT - 50	
♀ STARTING WEIGHT - 30	

SIDE CRUNCH

MAJOR MUSCLES IN USE:
External Oblique

STARTING POSITION:
- Lie on your side on the floor or on an abdominal bench with your head either level with or lower than your feet and your feet hooked under the leg pads.
- Your legs should be held straight or slightly bent.
- Hands can be crossed across the upper chest, positioned at the ears, or placed alongside the body.

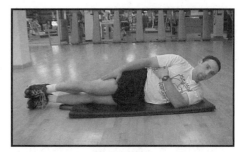

START

EXERCISE MOVEMENT:
- Begin the movement by lifting your shoulder off the floor (or bench) by curving your body upwards so that you are bending at your waist.
- You should finish the movement with your shoulder as high off the bench as possible.
- Return to the starting position by lowering your shoulders back down to the floor or bench.

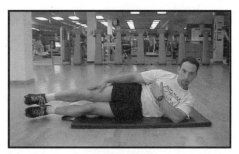

FINISH

EXERCISE TECHNIQUE POINTS:
- Do not bounce your torso off the bench or floor in order to complete the necessary repetitions.
- Do not allow your hips to lift off the bench in order to use that leverage to pull yourself up.
- You should not allow your torso to move forwards or backwards during the movement.

DIFFICULTY -	⊢⊣	⊢⊣
♂	STARTING WEIGHT - no weight	
♀	STARTING WEIGHT - no weight	

BALL SIDE CRUNCH

MAJOR MUSCLES IN USE:
External Oblique

STARTING POSITION:
- Lie on your side on top of an exercise ball and brace both feet against a wall or other sturdy object.
- Your legs should be slightly bent with one foot in front of the other.
- Hands can be crossed across the upper chest, positioned at the ears, or along side the body.

EXERCISE MOVEMENT:
- Begin the movement, lifting your shoulders upwards and away from the ball by curving your body so that you are bending to the side at your waist.
- You should finish with your shoulders as high off the ball as possible.
- Return to the starting position by lowering your shoulders back down towards the ball.

EXERCISE TECHNIQUE POINTS:
- Do not bounce your torso off the ball in order to complete the necessary repetitions.
- Do not allow your torso to rotate upwards as you lift your shoulders off the ball.
- You should not allow your torso to move forwards or backwards during the movement.

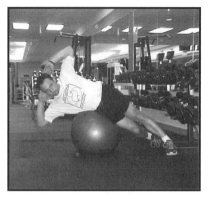

START

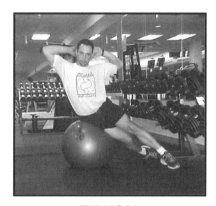

FINISH

DIFFICULTY -	H	H	H	H
♂ STARTING WEIGHT - no weight				
♀ STARTING WEIGHT - no weight				

OBLIQUE EXERCISES

HYPER-EXTENSION SIDE CRUNCH

MAJOR MUSCLES IN USE:
External Oblique

STARTING POSITION:
- Lie on the side of your hip on top of a hyper-extension bench and brace the sides of your ankles under the small pads that are now beside you. Your ankles should be located below the level of your hips.
- Your legs should be slightly bent with one foot in front of the other.
- Hands can be crossed across the upper chest, positioned at the ears or along side the body.

EXERCISE MOVEMENT:
- Begin the movement by lowering your shoulders down and towards the floor by curving your body so that you are bending to the side at your waist.
- You should finish with your shoulders as low as possible.
- Return towards the starting position by raising your shoulders up and away form the floor so that your upper body is almost perpendicular to the floor.

EXERCISE TECHNIQUE POINTS:
- Do not allow your torso to rotate upwards as you lift your shoulders up and away from the floor.
- You should not allow your torso to move forwards or backwards during the movement.
- To make the exercise more difficult you may wish to hang on to a weight as you perform the movement.

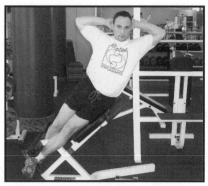
START

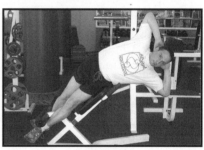
FINISH

DIFFICULTY -	H H H
♂ STARTING WEIGHT - no weight	
♀ STARTING WEIGHT - no weight	

BARBELL SIDE BENDS

MAJOR MUSCLES IN USE:
External Oblique

STARTING POSITION:
- Stand upright with your chest held high while you hold a barbell across the back of your shoulders.

EXERCISE MOVEMENT:
- Begin the movement by slowly bending to one side while keeping your back straight and your chest up.
- You should finish the movement with your torso bent to one side as far as is comfortable.
- Return to the starting position by bringing your torso back to an upright position.
- Repeat the same motion as outlined above for your other side.

EXERCISE TECHNIQUE POINTS:
- Do not lean forwards, backwards, or allow your body to rotate.
- Do not bounce at the end point.
- Do not bend so far to one side that you are uncomfortable.

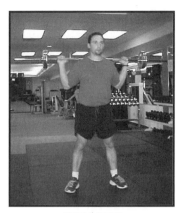

START

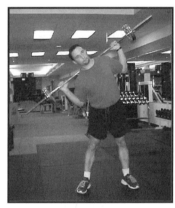

FINISH

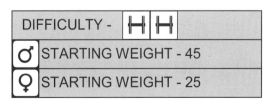

DIFFICULTY -	⊢⊢	
♂	STARTING WEIGHT - 45	
♀	STARTING WEIGHT - 25	

SINGLE SIDE BENDS

MAJOR MUSCLES IN USE:
External Oblique

STARTING POSITION:
- Stand upright with your chest held high. Hold one dumbbell beside your upper thigh with your palm facing inwards.

EXERCISE MOVEMENT:
- Begin the movement by slowly bending to the side that you are holding the dumbbell. Keep your arm straight and allow the dumbbell to slide down alongside your leg.
- You should finish the movement with your torso bent to one side as far as is comfortable.
- Return to the starting position by bringing your torso back to an upright stance.

EXERCISE TECHNIQUE POINTS:
- Do not lean forwards, backwards or allow your body to rotate as you bend to one side.
- Do not bounce at the end point.
- Do not bend so far to one side that you are uncomfortable.

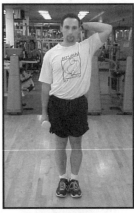

START

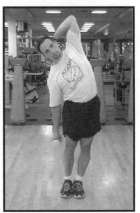

FINISH

DIFFICULTY -	┤├
♂ STARTING WEIGHT - 25	
♀ STARTING WEIGHT - 15	

CABLE SIDE BENDS

MAJOR MUSCLES IN USE:
External Oblique

STARTING POSITION:
- Stand with your body perpendicular to the pulley machine. Lean to your side and grasp the single handle that is attached to the cable with your closest hand. Your hand should be beside your upper thigh with your palm facing inwards.

EXERCISE MOVEMENT:
- Begin the movement by slowly bending to the opposite side while keeping your arm straight. Allow the handle to stay close to your body and slide alongside your leg.
- You should finish the movement with your torso bent to the opposite side as far as is comfortable.
- Return to the starting position by bringing your torso back to an upright position.

EXERCISE TECHNIQUE POINTS:
- Do not lean forwards, backwards, or allow your body to rotate.
- Do not bounce at the end point.
- Do not bend so far to one side that you are uncomfortable.
- Hold you chest high while performing the exercise.

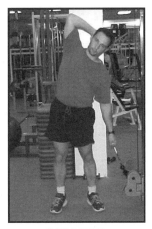

START

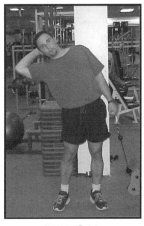

FINISH

DIFFICULTY -	⊢⊣	⊢⊣
♂	STARTING WEIGHT - 30	
♀	STARTING WEIGHT - 20	

OBLIQUE EXERCISES

INCLINE TWISTING LEG RAISE

MAJOR MUSCLES IN USE:
Rectus Abdominus, External Oblique

STARTING POSITION:
- Lie on an abdominal bench with your head higher than your feet. Steady your upper body by grabbing onto the end pads or available loops.
- Your knees should be bent at an angle of at least 90°. Cross your feet in order to keep your legs together during the exercise.

EXERCISE MOVEMENT:
- Begin the movement by curling your hips up and twisting them to one side as they rise off the incline bench. Your hips should follow an arc upwards with one side of your hips leading the motion.
- You should finish the movement with your thighs still perpendicular to the floor and your hips rotated so that one hip is closer to your shoulder than the other hip. If you find this too difficult, you can pull the knees in closer to the chest.
- Return to the starting position by reversing the motion.
- For the next repetition, follow the same procedure, but twist to the opposite side as you rise up.

EXERCISE TECHNIQUE POINTS:
- Do not bounce your hips off the bench to complete the necessary repetitions.
- Do not allow your knees to crossover the top of your head.
- The torso should curl or roll up and the back will round as you go from the starting position to the finish position.
- Keep your abdominal muscles tensed all the time in order to help control the twisting movement.

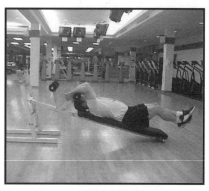

START

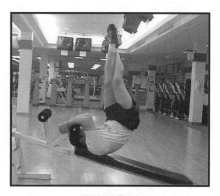

FINISH

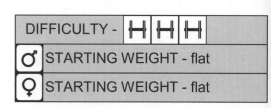

DIFFICULTY -	H	H	H
♂ STARTING WEIGHT - flat			
♀ STARTING WEIGHT - flat			

HANGING TWISTING LEG RAISE

MAJOR MUSCLES IN USE:
Rectus Abdominus, External Oblique

STARTING POSITION:
- You may perform this exercise in one of three different ways. You may hang from a bar with your hands about shoulder-width apart; or support yourself with your arms on dipping bars; or you may use a special upright leg raise machine.
- Your knees can be bent at any angle from 90° to just slightly bent. Cross your feet in order to help keep your legs together during the exercise.

EXERCISE MOVEMENT:
- Begin the movement by curling your hips upwards, allowing your legs to follow the motion of the hips. As you curl your hips in an arc upwards, lift one hip higher than the other so that one leg is over top of the other leg.
- You should finish the movement with your knees and feet held as high as possible with one leg on top of the other. Your upper body should still stay perpendicular to the floor. If you find this too difficult, you can pull the knees in closer to the chest.
- Return to the starting position by reversing the motion.

EXERCISE TECHNIQUE POINTS:
- Do not swing your legs in order to complete the necessary repetitions.
- Do not lift your legs with your knees straight.
- Allow your pelvis to tilt forward and to the side while you try to keep your feet as far away from your body as possible.

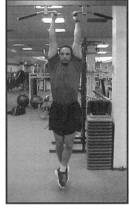

START

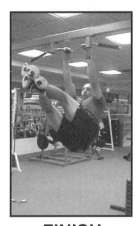

FINISH

DIFFICULTY -	H	H	H	H
♂ STARTING WEIGHT - bent knees				
♀ STARTING WEIGHT - bent knees				

OBLIQUE EXERCISES

LYING TWISTS

MAJOR MUSCLES IN USE:
External Oblique

STARTING POSITION:
- Lie on the floor with your legs straight up in the air, stabilize your upper body by stretching your arms out to your sides so that your upper body and arms resemble the letter "T".

EXERCISE MOVEMENT:
- Begin the movement by rotating your lower body so that both your legs move to one side as one hip rises off the floor.
- Finish the movement with your thighs touching the floor at one side of your body. Both your shoulders should remain on the floor.
- Return your legs to the starting position by reversing the motion by which you lowered them to one side. Continue the movement by moving your legs to the other side and repeating the motion.
- Return your legs back again to the starting position and repeat the entire movement for the desired number of repetitions.

EXERCISE TECHNIQUE POINTS:
- Do not bounce your knees and thighs off the floor in order to complete the necessary repetitions.
- Make sure that your shoulders stay on the ground as much as possible. If you lack flexibility, it is not unusual to have one shoulder come off the ground. However, try and focus on keeping your upper body as stable as possible.

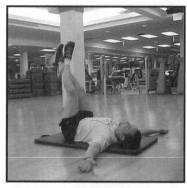

START

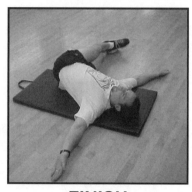

FINISH

DIFFICULTY -	H	H
♂ STARTING WEIGHT - no weight		
♀ STARTING WEIGHT - no weight		

OBLIQUE EXERCISES

BALL ROTARY TWISTS

MAJOR MUSCLES IN USE:
External Oblique

STARTING POSITION:
- Position your upper back and shoulders across the top of an exercise ball. Your feet should be flat on the floor and your hips, knees and shoulders should be in a straight line that is parallel to the floor.
- Grasp a dumbbell with both hands and position it straight above you.
- Your arms should be straight with your elbows locked.

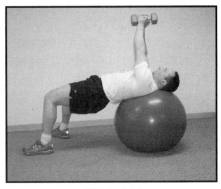

START

EXERCISE MOVEMENT:
- Begin by lower the dumbbell to one side along a semicircular path. Allow the ball to roll to the opposite side in order that you stay on top of the ball. Make sure your hips stay as level to the floor as possible.
- At the bottom portion of the movement your arms should be parallel to the floor.
- Reverse the motion by raising the dumbbell back along the same path that it was lowered.
- Repeat the same motion on the opposite side.

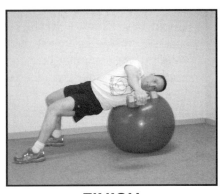

FINISH

EXERCISE TECHNIQUE POINTS:
- Do not bounce the dumbbell at the bottom of the movement.
- Do not bend your arms as you lower the weight to one side.
- Keep your abdominal and lower back muscles tensed to help you balance on the ball.
- Make sure that the dumbbell is positioned so that it is opposite your shoulders at all times.
- You may also choose to hang onto a weight plate instead of a dumbbell.

DIFFICULTY -	⊢ ⊢ ⊢ ⊢
♂ STARTING WEIGHT - 10	
♀ STARTING WEIGHT - 5	

OBLIQUE EXERCISES

HYPER-EXTENSION TWISTS

MAJOR MUSCLES IN USE:
External Oblique, Biceps Femoris, Semitendinosus, Semimembranosus, Gluteus Maximus, Erector Spinae

STARTING POSITION:
- Position your hips on the large pad of the hyperextension bench and the backs of your ankles under the small pads that are now behind you. Your ankles should be located slightly below your hips.
- Cross your hands over your chest or behind your head. Lock your knees.
- Your torso should be hanging downwards towards the floor.
- Tense the abdominal and lower back muscles.

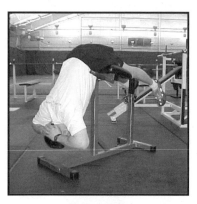

START

EXERCISE MOVEMENT:
- Begin by slowly raising your upper body, leading the movement with your chest and twisting your shoulders to one side so that one shoulder is higher than the other.
- Finish the exercise with your back slightly arched upwards, your torso slightly above parallel to the floor and one shoulder higher than the other.
- Lower yourself back to the starting position using the same twisting motion in reverse.
- As you repeat the motion, twist to the opposite side to work the other side of your midsection.

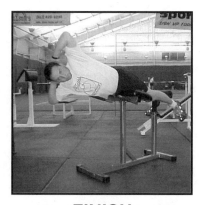

FINISH

EXERCISE TECHNIQUE POINTS:
- Make sure your back is always straight by keeping your chest up and your shoulders back.
- Do not bounce in the bottom position.
- Make sure you twist as much as possible as you raise your upper body.
- You may also make it more challenging by holding a weight to your chest or behind your head.

DIFFICULTY -	H	H
♂	STARTING WEIGHT - no weight	
♀	STARTING WEIGHT - no weight	

BALL HYPER-EXTENSION TWISTS

MAJOR MUSCLES IN USE:
External Oblique, Biceps Femoris, Gluteus Maximus, Erector Spinae

STARTING POSITION:
- Position your hips on top of an exercise ball and brace your feet against a wall or other study object.
- Cross your hands over your chest or behind your head. Lock your knees.
- Your torso should be hanging downwards across the ball towards the floor.
- Tense the abdominal and lower back muscles.

EXERCISE MOVEMENT:
- Begin by slowly raising your upper body, leading the movement with your chest and twisting your shoulders to one side so that one shoulder is higher than the other.
- Finish the exercise with your back slightly arched upwards, your torso slightly above parallel to the floor and one shoulder higher than the other.
- Lower yourself back to the starting position using the same twisting motion in reverse.
- As you repeat the motion, twist to the opposite side to work the other side of your midsection.

EXERCISE TECHNIQUE POINTS:
- Make sure your back is always straight by keeping your chest up and your shoulders back.
- Do not bounce in the bottom position.
- Make sure you twist as much as possible as you raise your upper body.
- You may also make it more challenging by holding a weight to your chest or behind your head.

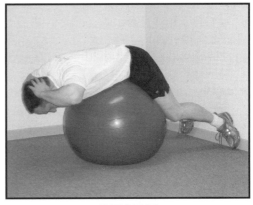

START

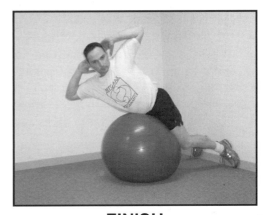

FINISH

DIFFICULTY -	H	H	H	H
♂	STARTING WEIGHT - no weight			
♀	STARTING WEIGHT - no weight			

TWISTING GOOD MORNINGS

MAJOR MUSCLES IN USE:
External Oblique, Erector Spinae, Biceps Femoris, Semitendinosus, Gluteus Maximus

STARTING POSITION:
- Position a barbell across the back of your shoulders.
- Feet should be shoulder width apart.
- Knees should be slightly bent.
- Shoulders are held back and your chest held high.
- Tense the abdominal and lower back muscles.

EXERCISE MOVEMENT:
- Begin by slowly bending forward, allowing your hips to lead the movement by moving them backwards first.
- End this lowering portion when your back is almost parallel to the floor.
- At this point reverse the movement by slowly raising your upper body, leading the movement with your chest and twisting your shoulders to one side so that one shoulder is higher than the other.
- Repeat the movement again when you are standing straight.

EXERCISE TECHNIQUE POINTS:
- Your back should always be straight. You can achieve this by keeping your chest up, your shoulders back and by pushing your buttocks out throughout the whole motion.
- Do not bounce in the bottom position.
- It is normal for your legs to bend slightly in the lowering portion.
- Make sure you keep your back straight by sticking the buttocks out throughout the whole motion.
- Try and twist as much as you can as you raise your upper body back to a standing position.

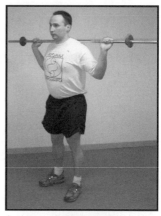

START

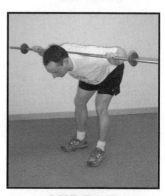

MIDDLE

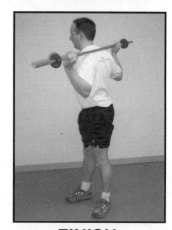

FINISH

DIFFICULTY -	H H H	
♂	STARTING WEIGHT - 45	
♀	STARTING WEIGHT - 25	

OBLIQUE EXERCISES

DUMBBELL TWISTING GOOD MORNINGS

MAJOR MUSCLES IN USE:
External Oblique, Erector Spinae, Biceps Femoris, Semitendinosus, Gluteus Maximus,

STARTING POSITION:
- Grasp a dumbbell with both hands and allow it to hang between your legs with your arms straight and feet spaced shoulder width apart.
- Knees should be slightly bent.
- Shoulders are held back and your chest held high.
- Tense the abdominal and lower back muscles.

EXERCISE MOVEMENT:
- Begin by slowly bending forward, allowing your hips to lead the movement by moving them backwards first.
- End this lowering portion when your back is almost parallel to the floor.
- At this point reverse the movement by slowly raising your upper body, leading the movement with your chest and twisting your shoulders to one side so that one shoulder is higher than the other.
- While keeping your arms straight, allow the dumbbell to rotate to one side as if you are pretending to throw the weight to one side and behind you.
- Once you are standing again, both feet should be on the floor pointing forward with your shoulders facing to one side and your arms straight in front of you holding the dumbbell at shoulder level.
- Lower the dumbbell to the floor by following the same motion as when you had lifted it. Repeat again on the opposite side.

EXERCISE TECHNIQUE POINTS:
- Your back should always be straight. You can achieve this by keeping your chest up, your shoulders back and by pushing your buttocks out throughout the whole motion.
- Do not bend both your arms.
- Make sure you keep your back straight by sticking the buttocks out throughout the whole motion.
- Try and twist as much as you can as you raise your upper body back to a standing position.
- Finish with the dumbbell held at shoulder level.

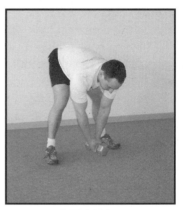

START

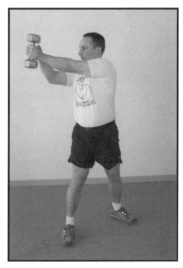

FINISH

DIFFICULTY -	H	H	H
♂ STARTING WEIGHT - 15			
♀ STARTING WEIGHT - 8			

OBLIQUE EXERCISES

STANDING CABLE TORSO ROTATIONS

MAJOR MUSCLES IN USE:
External Oblique

STARTING POSITION:
- Stand beside the pulldown machine at a distance of a little more than arms-length away with one of your shoulders facing the machine.
- Twist your upper body towards the machine while keeping your hips facing forward. Grasp one side of a rope handle from the high pulley with both hands. Place your feet shoulder width apart and tense your abdominal and lower back muscles.
- Your arms should be slightly bent.

EXERCISE MOVEMENT:
- While keeping your elbows locked at a slightly bent angle and the muscles in your midsection tensed, begin the exercise by rotating your torso across the front of your body towards the other side. Your hands should move along a semicircular path that is at a slight downwards angle towards the floor.
- At the end point in the movement your torso should be rotated as far as possible to the other side and facing away from the machine. Your hands should be at or just below shoulder level with your elbows slightly bent.
- Finish the exercise by returning the handle back to the starting position along the same path that it was moved.

EXERCISE TECHNIQUE POINTS:
- Remember to stand upright with your back straight and your chest held high.
- Do not allow your elbows to either straighten or bend more than 10° during any part of the motion.
- Do not twist the handle during any part of the movement.
- If you find it difficult to balance, place one foot slightly in front of the other and bend your knees.

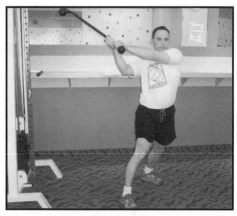

START

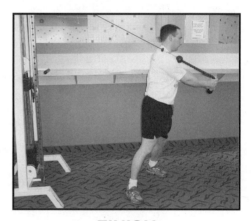

FINISH

DIFFICULTY -	H	H	H	
♂	STARTING WEIGHT - 20			
♀	STARTING WEIGHT - 15			

OBLIQUE EXERCISES

CALF EXERCISES

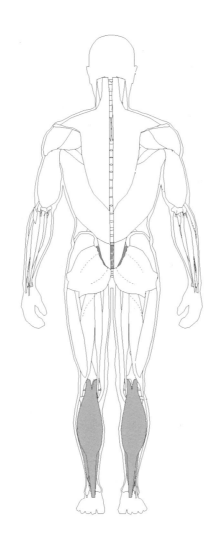

STANDING CALF RAISES

MAJOR MUSCLES IN USE:
Gastrocnemius, Soleus

STARTING POSITION:
- Place a barbell across the back of your shoulders.
- Your toes and the balls of your feet should be placed shoulder-width apart on a low platform. The arch of your foot should be right on the edge of the platform.
- Stand up straight while not allowing your lower back to arch inwards.

EXERCISE MOVEMENT:
- While keeping your legs as straight as possible, begin by lowering your heels so that you feel the calf muscles stretch. Your heels should go as far below the top of the platform as possible.
- Reverse the motion and rise up onto the balls of your feet and toes.
- At the top portion of the movement, you should be standing with all your weight on the balls of your feet and with your heels as high as possible.

EXERCISE TECHNIQUE POINTS:
- Make sure that the movement is straight up and down and that you are not rocking back and forth.
- Make sure you lower and raise your heels as much as possible since a full range of motion is the most effective method for developing the calf muscles.
- If you find it difficult to balance you may wish to use dumbbells instead of a barbell.

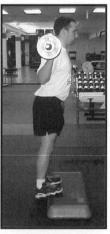

START

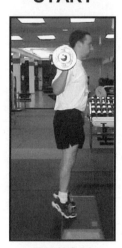

FINISH

DIFFICULTY -	H H H
♂ STARTING WEIGHT - 65	
♀ STARTING WEIGHT - 35	

SEATED CALF RAISES

MAJOR MUSCLES IN USE:
Soleus

STARTING POSITION:
- Sit at a seated calf raise machine or place a barbell across the tops of your thighs with your feet placed on a platform.
- Your toes and the balls of your feet should be placed shoulder width apart. The arch of your foot should be right on the edge of the platform.
- When using the machine, position the ends of your thighs (near your knees) under the pads and adjust the height so that your feet are parallel to the floor when your knees are firmly pressed against the pads.
- Sit up straight while not allowing your upper back to round.

EXERCISE MOVEMENT:
- Release the machine and begin the movement by lowering your heels so that you feel your calf muscles stretch. Your heels should be as far below the top of the platform as possible.
- When your heels are as far down as they will go, reverse the motion and begin to rise up onto the balls of your feet and toes.
- At the top portion of the movement, you should be supporting all the weight on the balls of your feet with your heels as high as possible.

EXERCISE TECHNIQUE POINTS:
- Make sure that the movement is straight up and down so that you are not rocking back and forth.
- Make sure you lower and raise your heels as much as possible since a full range of motion is the most effective method for developing the calf muscles.

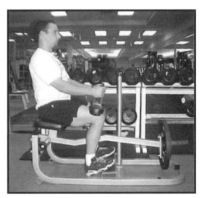

START

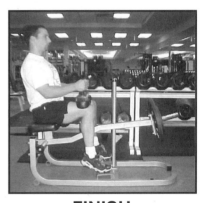

FINISH

DIFFICULTY - ꟼ⊢	
♂	STARTING WEIGHT - 75
♀	STARTING WEIGHT - 45

SINGLE LEG CALF RAISES

MAJOR MUSCLES IN USE:
Gastrocnemius, Soleus

STARTING POSITION:
- Hold the dumbbell at the side of the leg you plan to exercise.
- Place your toes and the ball of your foot on a step or platform about 4 – 6 inches high. The arch of your foot should be right on the edge of the step.
- Stand up straight while not allowing your lower back to arch inwards excessively. Tuck the non-exercising leg behind the exercising leg.

EXERCISE MOVEMENT:
- While keeping your leg as straight as possible, begin by lowering your heel so that you feel the muscles in your calf stretch. Your heel should be as far below the top of the step as possible.
- Reverse the motion and rise up onto the ball of your foot and toes.
- At the top portion of the movement you should be standing with all your weight on the ball of your foot with your heel as high as possible.

EXERCISE TECHNIQUE POINTS:
- Make sure that the movement is straight up and down and that you are not rocking back and forth.
- Make sure you lower and raise your heels as much as possible since a full range of motion is the most effective method for developing the calf muscles.

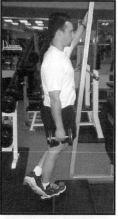
START

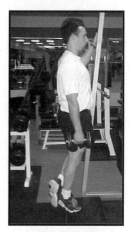
FINISH

DIFFICULTY -	⊢⊢	
♂	STARTING WEIGHT – no weight	
♀	STARTING WEIGHT – no weight	

TOE PRESSES

MAJOR MUSCLES IN USE:
Gastrocnemius, Soleus

STARTING POSITION:
- Position yourself in a leg press machine.
- Your toes and the balls of your feet should be placed shoulder width apart on the platform. The arch of your foot should be right on the edge of the platform.
- Straighten your legs to release the leg press while being careful not to allow your knees to lock completely.

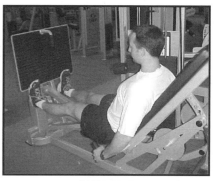

START

EXERCISE MOVEMENT:
- While keeping your legs as straight as possible, begin lowering the platform by bending your feet only at the ankles and bringing your toes towards you. You should feel your calf muscles stretch.
- Reverse the motion and push the platform back with the balls of your feet and toes.
- At the top portion of the movement, you should have all the weight on the balls of your feet with your toes pointed as much as possible away from you.

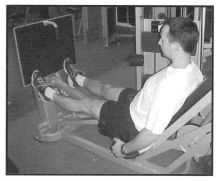

FINISH

EXERCISE TECHNIQUE POINTS:
- Make sure that you do not bounce in the bottom portion of the movement.
- Make sure you follow a full range of motion as possible since this is the most effective method for developing the calf muscles.
- Make sure that you do not bend at the knees at any point throughout the exercise.

DIFFICULTY -	⊢
♂ STARTING WEIGHT - 150	
♀ STARTING WEIGHT - 90	

CALF EXERCISES

SINGLE LEG TOE PRESS

MAJOR MUSCLES IN USE:
Gastrocnemius, Soleus

STARTING POSITION:
- Position yourself in a leg press machine.
- The toes and the ball of one foot should be placed near the edge of the platform and directly in line with your knee and hip. The arch of your foot should be right on the edge of the platform.
- Straighten your leg to release the leg press while not allowing your knee to lock completely.

EXERCISE MOVEMENT:
- While keeping your leg as straight as possible, begin lowering the platform by bending your foot only at the ankle and pulling your toes towards you. You should feel your calf muscles stretch.
- Reverse the motion and push back with the ball of your foot and your toes.
- At the top portion of the movement, you should have all the weight on the ball of your foot with your foot pointed away from you as much as possible.

EXERCISE TECHNIQUE POINTS:
- Make sure that you do not bounce in the bottom portion of the movement.
- Make sure you follow a full range of motion as possible as this is the most effective method for developing the calf muscles.
- Make sure you do not bend at the knee throughout the motion.

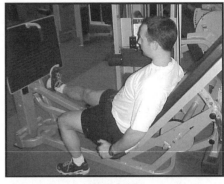

START

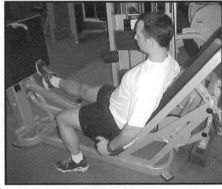

FINISH

DIFFICULTY -	⊢ ⊢	
♂	STARTING WEIGHT - 80	
♀	STARTING WEIGHT - 55	

CALF EXERCISES

DONKEY CALF RAISES

MAJOR MUSCLES IN USE:
Gastrocnemius, Soleus

STARTING POSITION:
- Position yourself in front of a stair case or calf raise machine so that your feet are on the step or platform and you are bent over at the waist, supporting yourself on another step, platform, or piece of equipment. Your back should be parallel to the ground.
- Your toes and the balls of your feet should be placed shoulder width apart on the bottom step or platform. The arch of your foot should be right on the edge of the step.

EXERCISE MOVEMENT:
- While keeping your legs as straight as possible, begin by lowering your heels so that you feel your calf muscles stretch. Your heels should be as far below the top of the step as possible.
- Reverse the motion and rise up onto the balls of your feet and toes.
- At the top portion of the movement, you should have all your weight on the balls of your feet with your heels up as high as possible.

EXERCISE TECHNIQUE POINTS:
- Make sure that the movement is straight up and down and that you are not rocking back and forth.
- Make sure to you lower and raise your heels as much as possible since a full range of motion is the most effective method for developing the calf muscles.
- Do not bounce or allow your knees to bend at any point in the movement.

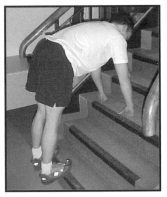

START

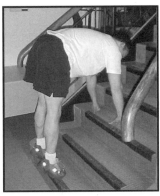

FINISH

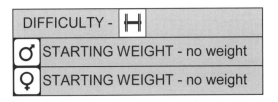

DIFFICULTY -	⊢⊣	
♂	STARTING WEIGHT - no weight	
♀	STARTING WEIGHT - no weight	

FRONT CALF EXERCISES

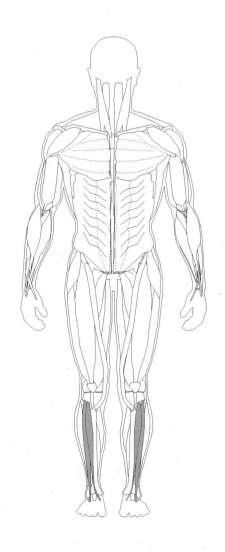

CABLE TOE PULLS

MAJOR MUSCLES IN USE:
Tibialis Anterior

STARTING POSITION:
- Position yourself seated in front of the low pulley of a cable machine.
- Secure the end of your foot to the cable by using an adjustable strap.
- Straighten your leg and allow your knee to completely lock and point your toes so that you feel a stretch along the front your calf.

EXERCISE MOVEMENT:
- While keeping your leg as straight as possible, begin by pulling the weight towards you by flexing your foot so that your toes point towards you and only your ankle moves.
- Reverse the motion by once again slowly pointing your toes.

EXERCISE TECHNIQUE POINTS:
- Make sure that you attach the loop to your foot securely.
- Keep your toes flexed upwards in order to help keep the loop on your foot.
- Make sure you follow a full range of motion as possible as this is the most effective method for developing the calf muscles.
- Make sure you do not bend at the knee at any point in the motion.

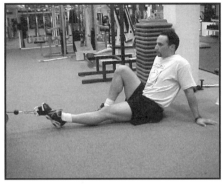

START

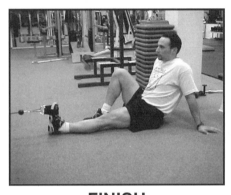

FINISH

DIFFICULTY -	H	H	
♂	STARTING WEIGHT - 45		
♀	STARTING WEIGHT - 25		

TOE RAISES

MAJOR MUSCLES IN USE:
Tibialis Anterior

STARTING POSITION:
- Position a barbell across your upper chest. Cross your arms across the bar to secure its position.
- The heels of your feet should be placed shoulder width apart on the platform. The arch of your foot should be right on the edge of the step.
- Stand up straight while not allowing your lower back to arch inwards.

EXERCISE MOVEMENT:
- While keeping your legs as straight as possible, begin by lowering your toes so that you feel the front of your calves stretch. Your toes should be as far below the top of the step as possible.
- Reverse the motion and shift your weight onto your heels by raising your toes as much as you can.
- At the top portion of the movement you should be standing with all your weight on your heels with your toes as high as possible.

EXERCISE TECHNIQUE POINTS:
- Make sure that the movement is straight up and down and that you are not rocking back and forth.
- A full range of motion is the most effective method for developing the calf muscles.
- Make sure you keep your legs completely straight and that your heels are firmly positioned on the platform.
- To help with balance, perform the exercise slowly and under control. You may also find it easier by holding dumbbells instead of a barbell.

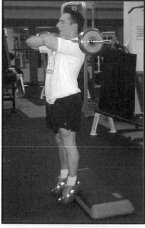

START

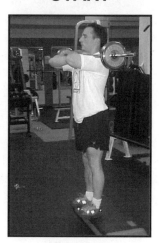

FINISH

DIFFICULTY -	H	H	H	
♂ STARTING WEIGHT - 65				
♀ STARTING WEIGHT - 35				

FOREARM EXERCISES

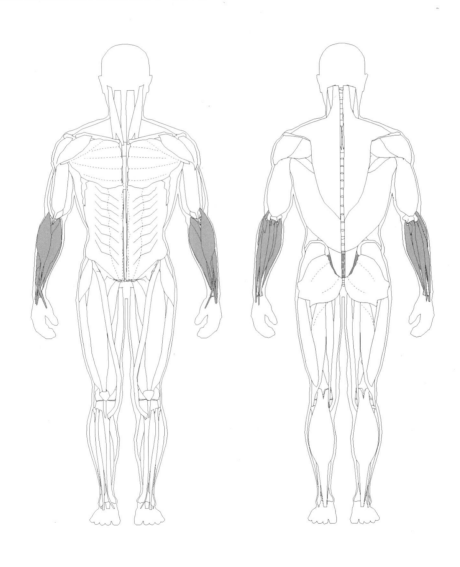

DUMBBELL WRIST CURLS

MAJOR MUSCLES IN USE:
Wrist Flexors

STARTING POSITION:
- Grasp a dumbbell with one hand using an underhand grip and place your forearm on a flat bench with your palm facing up.
- Allow your wrist and hand to extend off the edge of the bench while the rest of your forearm and elbow remains in contact with the bench.

EXERCISE MOVEMENT:
- With your wrist and hand extended off the edge of the bench, allow just your wrist to bend backwards and lower the dumbbell as far as possible.
- When your wrist has reached the endpoint of the range of motion, reverse the movement and raise the dumbbell back along the same path that it was lowered.
- Continue to lift the dumbbell as high as possible while only bending the wrist.

EXERCISE TECHNIQUE POINTS:
- Make sure that your elbow never comes off the bench while doing the exercise.
- Performing a full range of motion is the most effective method for developing the forearm muscles.

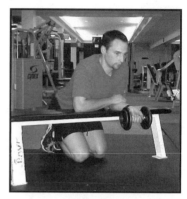

START

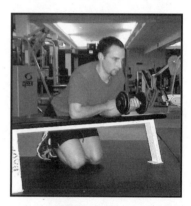

FINISH

DIFFICULTY -	⊢⊣
♂ STARTING WEIGHT - 20	
♀ STARTING WEIGHT - 10	

DUMBBELL WRIST EXTENSIONS

MAJOR MUSCLES IN USE:
Wrist Extensors

STARTING POSITION:
- Grasp a dumbbell with one hand using an overhand grip and place your forearm on a flat bench with your palm facing towards the floor.
- Allow your wrist and hand to extend off the edge of the bench, while the rest of your forearm and elbow remain in contact with the bench.

EXERCISE MOVEMENT:
- With your wrist and hand extended off the bench, allow just your wrist to bend and lower the dumbbell down as far as possible.
- When your wrist has reached the end point of the range of motion, reverse the movement and raise the dumbbell back along the same path that it was lowered.
- Continue to lift the dumbbell as high as possible while only bending at the wrist.

EXERCISE TECHNIQUE POINTS:
- Make sure that your forearm never comes off the bench while doing the exercise.
- Performing a full range of motion is the most effective method for developing the forearm muscles.

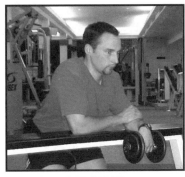

START

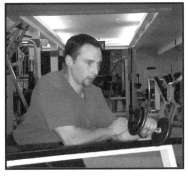

FINISH

DIFFICULTY -	H	
♂	STARTING WEIGHT - 15	
♀	STARTING WEIGHT - 8	

CABLE WRIST CURLS

MAJOR MUSCLES IN USE:
Wrist Flexors

STARTING POSITION:
- With both hands, grasp the short bar handle that is attached to the low pulley machine and place your forearms on your thighs (or a flat bench) with your palms facing upwards.
- Allow your wrist and hand to extend off of your knees or the edge of a bench, while the rest of your forearms and elbows remain in contact with the bench or your thighs.

EXERCISE MOVEMENT:
- Allow just your wrist to bend backwards and lower the bar as far as possible.
- When your wrist has reached the end point of the range of motion, reverse the motion and raise the bar back along the same path that it was lowered.
- Continue to lift the bar as high as possible while only bending at the wrist.

EXERCISE TECHNIQUE POINTS:
- Make sure that your forearms never come off the bench or your thighs while doing the exercise.
- Performing the full range of motion is the most effective method for developing the forearm muscles.

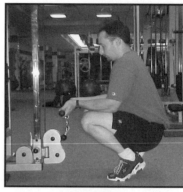
START

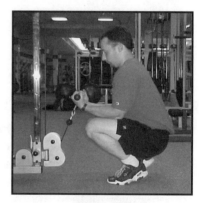
FINISH

DIFFICULTY - H H	
♂	STARTING WEIGHT - 40
♀	STARTING WEIGHT - 20

CABLE WRIST EXTENSIONS

MAJOR MUSCLES IN USE:
Wrist Extensors

STARTING POSITION:
- With both hands, grasp the short bar handle that is attached to the low pulley machine and place your forearms on your thighs or on a flat bench with your palms facing towards the floor.
- Allow your wrists and hands to extend off the edge of the bench or beyond your knees, while the rest of your forearms and elbows remain in contact with the bench or your thighs.

EXERCISE MOVEMENT:
- With your wrists and hands extended beyond the bench or your knee, allow just your wrist to bend and lower the bar down as far as possible.
- When your wrists have reached the end point of the range of motion, reverse the motion and raise the bar back along the same path that it was lowered.
- Continue to lift the bar as high as possible while only bending at the wrists.

EXERCISE TECHNIQUE POINTS:
- Make sure that your forearms never come off the bench or your thighs while doing the exercise.
- Performing the full range of motion is the most effective method for developing the forearm muscles.

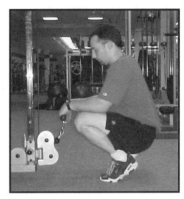

START

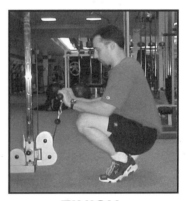

FINISH

DIFFICULTY - H H		
♂	STARTING WEIGHT - 30	
♀	STARTING WEIGHT - 15	

REVERSE CURLS

MAJOR MUSCLES IN USE:
Biceps Brachii, Brachialis, Wrist Extensors

STARTING POSITION:
- Stand with knees slightly bent and feet about shoulder width apart.
- Arms hang straight at your sides with the bar resting on your upper thighs.
- Use an overhand grip on the bar.

EXERCISE MOVEMENT:
- While keeping your upper arms stationary, begin by bending at the elbows and lifting the weight up following the natural curve of your arm movement.
- At midpoint in the motion, your elbows should be bent at 90° with your forearms parallel to the floor and your upper arms perpendicular to the floor.
- Finish with the barbell at shoulder level with your upper arms remaining perpendicular to the floor.
- Return the weight to the starting position while not allowing your elbows to move backwards.
- Before beginning another repetition, your arms should once again be straight.

EXERCISE TECHNIQUE POINTS:
- Do not sway your torso back and forth.
- Do not allow your elbows to move back and forth as you lift the weight.
- Maintain good posture with your back straight at all times.
- Do not bend your knees or "jump" the weight up to complete a repetition.
- You may wish to use an E-Z curl bar to reduce the strain on the wrists.

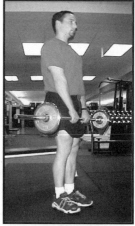

START

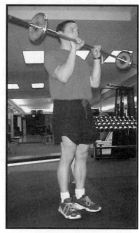

FINISH

DIFFICULTY -	⊢	
♂	STARTING WEIGHT - 40	
♀	STARTING WEIGHT - 20	

BEHIND-THE-BACK WRIST CURLS

MAJOR MUSCLES IN USE:
Wrist Flexors

STARTING POSITION:
- Place a barbell behind your thighs and grasp the bar with an underhand grip and your palms facing away from you.
- Straighten your arms, lock your elbows, and allow your wrist to straighten.

EXERCISE MOVEMENT:
- With your hands hanging straight down, allow just your wrists to bend upwards and raise the barbell as high as possible in a path away from your body.
- When you have raised the bar as high as possible, reverse the motion and lower the dumbbell back along the same path that it was raised.

EXERCISE TECHNIQUE POINTS:
- Make sure that your elbows are locked and that you do not bend at the elbow.
- Performing the full range of motion is the most effective method for developing the forearm muscles, so try to raise the bar as high as possible.
- Do not allow your heels to come off the ground in order to "jump" the weight up to complete the repetition.

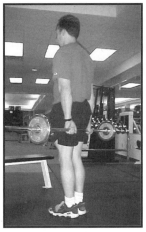

START

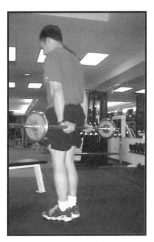

FINISH

DIFFICULTY - H		
♂	STARTING WEIGHT - 45	
♀	STARTING WEIGHT - 25	

FOREARM EXERCISES 341

STRAIGHT ARM WRIST EXTENSION

MAJOR MUSCLES IN USE:
Wrist Extensors

STARTING POSITION:
- Place a barbell in front of your thighs and grasp the bar with both hands in an overhand grip with your palms facing towards you.
- Straighten your arms and lock your elbows and allow your wrists to straighten.

EXERCISE MOVEMENT:
- With your arms and hands hanging straight down, allow just your wrists to bend upwards and raise the barbell as high as possible in a semicircular path away from your body.
- When you have raised the bar as high as possible, reverse the motion and lower the barbell back along the same path that it was raised.

EXERCISE TECHNIQUE POINTS:
- Make sure that your elbows are locked and that you do not bend them at any point during the exercise.
- Performing the full range of motion is the most effective method for developing the forearm muscles, so remember to raise the bar as high as possible.
- Do not allow your heels to come off the ground in order to "jump" the weight up to complete the repetition.

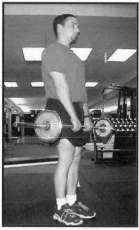

START

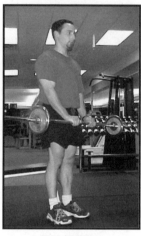

FINISH

DIFFICULTY -	⊢⊣	⊢⊣
♂ STARTING WEIGHT - 35		
♀ STARTING WEIGHT - 20		

FOREARM EXERCISES

INDEX